UNSAFE ABORTION AND WOMEN'S HEALTH

Unsafe Abortion and Women's Health

Change and Liberalization

COLIN FRANCOME
Middlesex University, UK

Routledge
Taylor & Francis Group
LONDON AND NEW YORK

First published 2015 by Ashgate Publishing

2 Park Square, Milton Park, Abingdon, Oxfordshire OX14 4RN
52 Vanderbilt Avenue, New York, NY 10017

Routledge is an imprint of the Taylor & Francis Group, an informa business

First issued in paperback 2020

British Library Cataloguing in Publication Data
A catalogue record for this book is available from the British Library

The Library of Congress has cataloged the printed edition as follows:
Francome, Colin.
Unsafe abortion and women's health : change and liberalization / by Colin Francome.
pages cm
Includes bibliographical references and index.
ISBN 978-1-4724-2761-8 (hardback)
1. Abortion. 2. Abortion – Law and legislation.
3. Birth control. I. Title.

HQ767.F7198 2014
362.1988'8–dc23

2013049432

ISBN 978-1-4724-2761-8 (hbk)
ISBN 978-0-367-59918-8 (pbk)

Contents

List of Tables *vii*
Preface *ix*
Acknowledgements *xi*
List of Abbreviations *xiii*

1 Introduction 1

2 Europe 19

3 Asia 53

4 Africa 93

5 Latin America and the Caribbean 133

6 Oceania 169

7 North America 177

8 Conclusions and Recommendations 191

Bibliography *203*
Index *221*

List of Tables

1.1 Unmet need, met need and total demand for family planning (FP) 2
1.2 The number of abortions by region 3
2.1 Average number of births in 2013 19
2.2 Maternal and infant mortality rates 20
2.3 Maternal and infant mortality rates Southern and Western Europe 21
2.4 Romania: percentage of pregnancies ending in abortion (excluding foetal deaths and miscarriage 41
2.5 Abortions and births in Russia 43
2.6 Abortions and births in Sweden 47
2.7 Abortions and births in Ukraine 48
3.1 Eastern and Southern Asia 54
3.2 South Central and Western Asia 55
4.1 Eastern and Middle African Countries 95
4.2 Northern, Southern and Western Africa 96
5.1 The 29 countries of Latin America and the Caribbean (2011) 135
6.1 Oceania: maternal and infant mortality 169

Preface

In 2008 it was estimated that 47,000 women died of unsafe abortions which is one death in every eleven minutes.

Unsafe abortion is largely a problem of poverty. Most women in rich countries can obtain safe abortions locally and others can travel to countries where abortion is safe. In contrast, poor people have to face the vagaries of abortions occurring outside safe, legal health services. This leads to 99 per cent of abortion deaths occurring in poor countries.

Apart from the women who die there are numerous others who suffer illness.

There are those following religious doctrine who believe abstinence is the answer to unwanted pregnancies. However, country by country evidence provided in this book has yet to find a country where such a policy has proved effective.

Official figures suggest over four times as many women died from unsafe abortion as were killed in all the terrorist attacks around the world. Yet, while terrorism dominates the media and billions are spent hoping to prevent it, unsafe abortion remains the silent killer.

The evidence shows that the countries with the lowest rates of abortion are the Western European ones with legal operations backed up by good quality sex education and contraception.

The Guttmacher Institute reported that over 200 million women were sexually active, not wanting a pregnancy, yet not using contraception.

It is time to put women's health before religious dogma and to provide safe legal abortions worldwide.

Acknowledgements

Special thanks to Stan Henshaw of the Guttmacher Institute who wrote most of the US chapter, commented on the other chapters and provided the Appendix to Chapter 7.

Many others helped with this book. They include: Wendy Savage of Doctors for Free Choice on Abortion; Louise Bury of Marie Stopes International; Carla Francome; Martin Clough and Dr Marion Newman.

List of Abbreviations

AP	Associated Press
BPAS	British Pregnancy Advisory Service
CAWN	Central American Women's Network
CEDAW	Committee on the Elimination of Discrimination against Women
Can	Catholic News Agency
COPUA	Coalition for the Prevention of Unsafe Abortion
CRR	Centre for Reproductive Rights
	International Campaign for Women's Rights to Safe Abortion (sometimes ICWRSA)
IJFP	International Journal of Family Planning
IPPF	International Planned Parenthood Federation
IRIN	Integrated Regional Information Networks
MSI	Marie Stopes International
MVA	Manual Vacuum Aspiration
PI	Pathfinder International
PRI	Population Research Institute
WHO	World Health Organization
WOW	Women on Waves

Chapter 1
Introduction

'Restrictive laws do not reduce the abortion rate they merely result in women dying'
Dr Dorothy Shaw

Women in the richer countries of the world have access to safe abortions either in their own countries or as with Ireland, in a nearby country. In contrast, women in the developing countries face unsafe operations. We can be grateful for the fact that abortion deaths have declined somewhat. In 2008 there were an estimated 47,000 abortion deaths which is a reduction from the 2003 figure of 56,000. Hopefully the growth in availability of misoprostol and mifepristone will further reduce the figure. However, we can still agree with the comments from an article published by the World Health Organization (WHO) that 'Unsafe abortion remains one of the most neglected sexual and reproductive health problems' (Grimes et al. 2006) This book aims to raise the importance of the issue and to propose measures to reduce the number of maternal deaths.

Latest figures indicate that nearly half the abortions in the world are unsafe and that nearly all (98 per cent) of unsafe abortions occur in the developing countries. In the developing world 56 per cent of abortions are unsafe compared with six per cent in the developed world (Guttmacher Institute 2013). The world figures showed a marked reduction in the incidence of abortions towards the beginning of the century. The number of abortions declined from 35 per 1,000 women of child bearing age in 1995 to 29 in 2003. However, by 2008 the rate had only fallen marginally to 28. The proportion of abortions that occur in the developing world increased between 1995–2008 from 78 per cent to 86 per cent. This was in part because the proportion of women living in the developing world increased. Consequently, while the number of abortions in the developed countries decreased by 600,000 between 2003–2008 in the developed world, they increased by 2.8 million in the developing world (Guttmacher Institute 2013). Apart from the women who die of abortion there are numerous others who suffer illness. The World Health Organization (WHO) estimates that around 20–30 per cent of women having an unsafe abortion suffer reproductive tract infections. The result is that around two per cent of women become infertile due to unsafe abortion and five per cent suffer chronic infection (Grimes et al. 2006).

In contrast to the situation in many of the poorer countries, legal abortion is now available in all industrialized countries except Ireland, Malta and Poland. National Health Insurance also covers the procedure in most industrialized countries. Abortion is still highly restricted in most countries of Latin America and Africa and in parts of Asia. Worldwide, the trend toward relaxing restrictions has continued.

Contraception

The Guttmacher Institute states that 215 million women worldwide are sexually active, do not want a pregnancy, but not using modern methods of contraception. It continued to say that making contraception available to all these women would only result in a cost of four billion dollars. This is roughly the cost of two weeks military operations in Afghanistan (Kristof 2012).

The concept of an unmet need for contraception has been used by the international population community since the 1960s. It developed out of surveys which showed education deficiencies with a great lack of knowledge, attitudes and practices (KAP) about contraception. The fertility surveys found a gap between what people knew their fertility preferences to be and their actions to achieve their desires. Further research in over 75 countries by the Demographic and Health Surveys (DHS) programmes provided further information. The unmet need for contraception is defined as the proportion of currently sexually active women who do not want any more children at present but are not using any form of family planning. There are a variety of reasons why women who do not wish to become pregnant nevertheless do not use contraception. These include opposition from sexual partner, concern about real or imagined side effects, lack of knowledge or lack of finance. When I conducted research into why women in the US, Ireland and the UK did not use contraception despite not wishing a pregnancy, I found the most quoted reasons for not use of contraception was 'had intercourse unexpectedly'.

Table 1.1 Unmet need, met need and total demand for family planning (FP)

	Unmet need	Met need	Total demand for FP	Percentage of demand satisfied
East Europe and Central Asia	13	60	73	82
East Asia and Pacific	14	57	71	80
South Asia	20	47	67	70
Latin America and the Caribbean	17	63	80	79
Middle East and North Africa	11	57	68	84
Sub-Saharan Africa	26	25	51	49

Source: World Bank 2013, p. 6. As this report is used so much it is not routinely referenced in subsequent chapters.

Using data from international surveys taken between 2000 and 2009 we can look at regional differences in met and unmet need for contraception.

The results show that sub-Saharan Africa has both the highest unmet need for contraception and the lowest percentage of the demand satisfied. This fact will account in part for the demand for abortion and also for the preparedness for good quality child care. In the forthcoming country by country analysis I include the data for the percentage of contraceptive prevalence for numerous countries. It is based on use of all methods traditional and modern. It identifies the percentage of women of reproductive age – here taken as 15–49 years and not 15–44 which is sometimes used especially for abortion analysis. It is measured for married women or those living with a partner (WHO 2012).

The Number of Abortions Safe and Unsafe

The number of abortions worldwide can be seen in Table 1.2.

Table 1.2 The number of abortions by region

	Number of abortions	Abortion rate per 1,000 age 15–44	Percentage unsafe
Europe	4.2	27	9%
Asia	27.3	28	40%
Africa	6.4	29	97%
Latin America	4.4	32	95%
North America	1.4	19	1% (my estimate)
Oceania	0.1	17	15%
World	43.8	28	49%

Source: Sedge et al., Guttmacher Institute 2013. Figures refer to 2008.

The table shows the worldwide number of abortion is estimated at nearly 44 million. Which is a slight increase on figures for 2003 but below the estimates for 1995. The highest overall rate is in Latin America with a rate of 32/1000 women age 15–44 and the lowest is Oceania with an abortion rate of 17. The estimate is that the world rate is 28 per 1,000 and that 14 per 1,000 are safe and almost an equal number unsafe (also 14 per 1,000).

Amongst the developed countries there has been a fall in the number of abortions from 10.0 million in 1995 to 6.6 million in 2003 and 6.0 million in 2008. The rate per 1,000 women at risk (aged 15–44) has also declined from 39 in 1995 to 24 in 2008. This is almost a 40 per cent reduction.

Amongst the developing countries the situation is more blurred. The absolute number of abortions has increased from 35.5 million in 1995 to 37.8 million in 2008. However, this is largely due to growth in population and their abortion rate as measured per woman at risk shows a reduction from 34 per 1,000 in 1995 to 29 in 2008.

The regional analysis of the number of unsafe abortions shows that unsafe abortions are concentrated in Africa, Latin America and parts of Asia. The Asian figure would be much higher were it not for China.

Further investigation of the European situation reveals great differences which will be more fully discussed in the next chapter. In Western Europe the abortion rate is only 12/1,000. In Eastern Europe it is the very high figure of 43/1000 which is over three times the Western European level (Guttmacher Institute 2013)

The Pro-life Position

There are those who take the position that the law should proscribe abortion on the grounds that life begins at conception and that society should protect life. The major organizations will oppose abortion where a woman has been impregnated following rape. We shall see that these groups have had some success in maintaining restrictive laws especially in the poorer countries. However, there are a number of points to be made. First, life does not begin at conception. It begins before conception as it is necessary to have a live sperm and a live egg. A second point is that 'pro-life' groups are largely opposed to many pro-life activities such as artificial insemination by donor (AID) or *in-vitro* fertilization (IVF). These developments have helped thousands of women to have children they would otherwise have been denied.

A third important question is whether it is possible to legislate to create an abortion-free society. The country by country analysis in this book shows that in every country without legal abortion there is evidence of women having illegal and often unsafe abortions, or travelling to have abortions in a different country. Countries such as Holland and Switzerland have relatively few abortions by having good quality contraception.

Abortion is a reality

The fact that this book identifies abortion as being used by women in all countries suggests that it cannot be eliminated by authorities keeping it illegal. The implication is that governments can only pass laws which will decide whether abortions are safe and legal or unsafe and illegal. We will see that in countries such as the United States and Britain a great number of abortions occurred even when abortion was illegal. Dr Dorothy Shaw, the president of the International Federation of Gynaecologists and Obstetricians (FIGO) speaking at a WHO forum in December 2006, stated that evidence on sex and reproductive health 'clearly shows the continuing track record of preventable deaths and illness in catastrophic numbers that would not be tolerated in most other imaginable situations'. She continued to say that sexual and reproductive rights are integral parts of basic human rights and that 'restrictive laws do not reduce the abortion rate, they merely result in woman dying (WHO Forum 2006).

It is relatively rare for countries to legalize abortion and then to make it illegal. However, Romania provides an example of the problems that can follow. In 1965, it had a birth rate of 14.6 per thousand population and 64 abortion deaths. In 1966 it restricted abortion rights and access to contraception. The birth rate almost doubled to 27.4 in 1967 and the number of abortion deaths rose to 170 which is almost three times the 1965 level. Then, in subsequent years the number of abortion deaths continued to rise and were 364 in 1971 which is over five times its earlier level and the birth rate in that year was down to 19.1 and approaching its earlier level (Francome 1976).

If abortion is not readily and legally accessible, poorer women will be forced to seek treatment from local operators with potentially disastrous results. However, richer women will become abortion 'tourists'. In the early part of the twentieth century British women went to France for abortions. When British law was changed French women began travelling to Britain in great numbers. In the early 1960s Swedish women went to Poland and women from the US went to Britain. After the legalization of abortion in New York in 1970, Canadian women went to the US. When financial restrictions were placed on poorer women in the US they began to travel to Mexico. German and Belgian women went to Holland until a change in their law. In Britain in 1972, over 50,000 women from overseas had abortions in the country and there was a spectacular growth in the number of Spanish women until its law changed. In 2006, Swedish operators expressed a willingness to help their Polish neighbours who had earlier helped their women obtain treatment. Irish women still travel to Britain, even from Northern Ireland where the 1967 Abortion Act does not apply. Over the years there have been distinct patterns where women travel abroad for abortions, but simultaneously, activists are working to change the law in their home country.

The International Conference on Population and Development of 1994 drew attention to the high levels of maternal mortality and a target was set to halve the 1990 rates by the year 2,000 and halve it again by the year 2015 (UN 2004).

Need for worldwide change

As recently as the 1960s there were only a few places in the world such as the Soviet Union which had liberal abortion laws. When the British Abortion Act 1967 came into operation on 27 April 1968 with no residential requirement, it meant that affluent women from all over the world could have access to safe legal abortions. It was followed by a great change in laws in other countries. In the period until 1982 twelve countries passed laws to allow abortion on request. These were Austria, Denmark, France, German Democratic Republic, Holland, Italy, Norway, Singapore, Slovenia, Sweden, Tunisia, United States and Yugoslavia.

In addition, 26 countries extended their grounds but did not officially give the right to choose. These were Australia, Belize, Canada, Chile, Cyprus, El Salvador, Fiji, Finland, Germany Federal Republic, Greece, Guatemala, Hong Kong, Iceland, India, Israel, Korea (Republic of), Kuwait, Luxembourg, Morocco, New Zealand, Peru, Seychelles, South Africa, United Arab Emirates and Zimbabwe. Chile and El Salvador have since eliminated all grounds for abortion and therefore move in the opposite direction.

Countries providing women with the right to choose, or at least obtain, abortion on a wide variety of grounds were predominantly the wealthier ones. In recent years there have been further changes. In 1995 the Beijing Platform for Action called on governments to rescind restrictive abortion laws that were punitive to women and from then until 2013, the following countries liberalized their laws: Albania (1996), Benin (2003), Bhutan (2004) Burkina Faso (1996), Cambodia (1997), Chad (2002), Columbia (2006), Ethiopia (2004), Guinea (2000), Guyana (1995), Mali (2002), Nepal (2002), Portugal (2007), St Lucia (2004), South Africa (1996), Swaziland (2005), Switzerland (2002) and Togo (2007) (Katzive 2007, Centre for Reproductive Rights 2007) Kenya (2010), Uruguay (2012), Ireland (marginally) (2013). In April 2007, Mexico City passed a law allowing abortion on request in the early part of pregnancy and Victoria State in Australia did so in 2008 (Henshaw, personal communication 2013).

Children Born into Poverty

There is a very high correlation with high family size and poverty for children. Niger is a good example. The country had the highest fertility rate in the world at 7.5 per woman (2011). It also has high infant mortality at 110 per 1,000 in 2011. This means that for every 100 fertile women in the country there will be an average of 825 infant deaths before the age of one year. Others will die later in childhood. The suffering that this waste of life causes can only be imagined as women and their partners are clearly unable to care for their children adequately. Furthermore, there will be many other children who survive, but who do so without proper nutrition, health and social care. The introduction of proper facilities for contraception and abortion, especially as part of a wider programme to improve medical and social support, could prevent much misery amongst poor women who have to face bringing children into the world without adequate resources.

Other countries are in a similar position. Women in Timor Leste, Afghanistan, Guinea-Bissau and Uganda all had an average family size of over seven children per woman during the period 2000–05. Other countries such as Mali, Burundi, Liberia, Angola and the Democratic Republic of the Congo had a fertility rate of over six children per woman. All these also have high rates of ill health amongst both women and children. Overall, in the poor countries 170 million children are underweight and over three million of these children die each year as a result (Wright 2006, p. 485). Access to modern contraceptives and abortion facilities are part of a wider need to improve maternal and children's health We can see that things have improved, but there is still a long way to go.

International Developments in Aid for Family Planning

Official Norwegian development assistance began in 1952 and an emphasis on family planning followed in 1966. One point that was mentioned by experts was that population growth was hampering economic growth. In 1968 the Norwegian parliament decided that family planning should be a priority for development assistance. Norad, the government development agency allocated ten per cent of bilateral development assistance to family planning in 1970. In the following year parliament supported Norad's policy proposal of placing family planning as part of primary care with the aim of helping to improve the health of women and their children (Austveg and Sundby 2005). The importance of contraception and reproductive health to development was also recognized in 1989 at a conference in Amsterdam, which placed as a target developed countries providing four per cent of their Overseas Development Aid to population activities.

At the International Conference on Population and Development (ICPD) in 1994, Norway produced a report stressing 'the seriousness of present population growth and the need to counteract the negative effects on the environment'. According to Population Action International, Norway was the only country before 1994 to allocate at least four per cent of overseas development assistance to population. Norway has been one of the largest donors to UNFPA since its inception in 1969 and also a large donor to IPPF. Overall, the proportion of family planning aid in 2004 for all donors was 5.5 per cent and so the 1994 target has been achieved. However, in 2004 in several countries the percentage was below two per cent. These were Austria (0.5 per cent), Italy (1.0 per cent), Greece (1.4 per cent), Spain (1.5 per cent) and Germany (1.9 per cent). So improved contributions from these countries would be useful in an area where funds are short. Countries above the five per cent level included Netherlands (10.2 per cent) US (9.2 per cent) UK (8.4 per cent) and Sweden (7.2 per cent).

The 1994 ICPD in Cairo led to the first major international agreement on unsafe abortion with 180 countries agreeing a programme of action. Its proposals fell short of deciding that a woman should have the right to choose in the early months of pregnancy. However, it drew attention to the public impact of unsafe abortion and the need to expand family planning services to reduce the recourse to abortion. In paragraph 7.2 it stated:

> Reproductive rights ... rest on the recognition of the basic right of all couples and individuals to decide freely and responsibly the number, spacing and timing of their children and to have the information and means to do so, and the right to attain the highest standard of sexual and reproductive health. It also includes their right to make decisions concerning reproduction free of discrimination, coercion and violence, as expressed in human rights documents. (Hessini 2005)

Hessini assessed how the principles and recommendations of the conference have been applied to increasing women's access to 'affordable, safe and legal abortion services' in the decade until 2004. She asserted that studies have increased the knowledge of the magnitude of unsafe abortion, that they have raised the awareness of women's experience of illegal abortion and linked it to other public health and women's rights issues. This drew attention to the fact that there have been several studies of abortion complications. For example, one study estimated that over

20,000 women were being treated for abortion-related illness in Kenyan public hospitals. We will be providing similar evidence from a variety of countries.

It also stated that women still face numerous barriers in countries where abortion is legal. For example, in India where abortion has been legal for over thirty years, 76 per cent of facilities were not licensed and 68 per cent of providers were not registered. The quality of services can be problematical and a study in Tamil Nadu, India found that close to 30 per cent of women seeking legal abortions experienced moderate to serious post-abortion complications. There is evidence of improvement since that time and the quality of care in India seems to be improving as we will discuss.

The Millennium Development Goals grew out of the United Nations Millennium Declaration adopted by 189 member states in 2000. There were eight goals. Three of them were directly related to reproductive health. As mentioned earlier, it aimed to reduce the maternal mortality ratio by three quarters and the under-fives mortality rate by two thirds between 1990 and 2015. A third goal was to have halt the spread of AIDS and to reverse it by the year 2015. Other goals were to eradicate extreme poverty and hunger, promote gender equality and empower women and ensure environment sustainability (WHO 2005).

At the 2005 World Summit, leaders committed themselves to 'achieving universal access to reproductive health by 2015' as set out by the International Conference on Population and Development. This aim was to be integrated into strategies to attain the internationally agreed development goals including those contained in the millennial declaration aimed at reducing maternal mortality, improving maternal health, reducing child mortality, improving gender equality, combating HIV/AIDS and eradicating poverty (RF News 2007). If this occurs then we would also expect the number of unsafe abortions to be reduced.

World Fertility Rates

The world fertility rate has been declining. In 1970–75 it was 4.5 children per woman. This had declined to 3.0 in 1990: 95m to 2.8 from 1995–2000 and 2.5 in 2011 (CIA 2012, p. 807). Amongst the more developed regions fertility has been much lower than average. In the years 1970–75, it was 2.1 children per woman but had declined to 1.6 in the period 1995–2000. In the less developed regions fertility was 5.4 children per woman in 1970–75 and had declined by over two children per woman by 1995–2000 when the average had reduced to an average of 3.1 children per woman. However, it is the poorest women who have the highest birth rate. In the countries designated by the UN as the least developed regions the birth rate has not fallen so fast. In 1970–75 it was 6.6 children per woman and had declined by one child per woman to 5.5 in 1995–2000. So more children are born to these women in poverty, where there are also the higher rates of infant deaths (UN 2004, p. 29).

Within these overall figures there are some countries which have greatly decreased their birth rate. In Iran there was an average of 6.4 children per woman in 1964 but by 1996 it had reduced by nearly four children to 2.5 per woman. Similarly, in Brazil the average woman had 5.7 children in 1965 and the number fell to 2.3 in 1996 (UN 2004). So rapid changes may occur and it is feasible that poor countries could make significant strides in a short time.

Costs of Restrictive Laws

Hessini also drew attention to the fact that restrictive laws, unsafe abortions and poor standards of care lead to higher costs in some respects. Using data from Africa, a model showed that treating incomplete abortions in hospitals costs around ten times the cost of providing safe legal abortions in a primary health centre. Costs are also reduced where Manual Vacuum Aspiration (MVA) is used instead of Dilation and Curettage (D&C). In 1995 the Fourth World Conference on Women called for governments to 'review laws containing punitive measures against women who have undergone illegal abortions'.

There have been a number of other important events, including a 2003 Conference in Ethiopia discussing unsafe abortion in Africa and in 2004, a South African Conference on the role of medical abortion in expanding women's access to safe treatment (Hessini 2005, p. 91).

International organizations have also taken an increased role. One such is the Committee on the Elimination of Discrimination against Women (CEDAW). This group points out that neglecting health care specific to women is a form of sex discrimination which Governments are obliged to remedy.

Abortion as a Controversial Issue

Passions often run high when debating the issue. Those of us who support a woman's right to choose point to the dangers of illegal abortion. We also draw attention to the fact that if women are forced to bear children for whom they cannot care properly, then it can lead to social problems. Opponents of choice may point to the rights of the foetus to be born They may also argue that legalizing abortion may lead to a decline in morals. However, this book will agree strongly with the view put forward in Boston (US) by the Catholic priest Robert Drinan. This is that the fact that some people believe abortion to be wrong should not impinge on the quality of care for those who do not share that view (Francome 1984, pp. 112–13).

Major Religions and Abortion

In 2009, Christianity made up a third (33.4 per cent) of the world's population with one in six (16.8 per cent) people worldwide practising this faith. Muslims made up just over one in five (22.4 per cent) and they were divided between Shiite and Sunni Muslims. The third biggest group were Hindus, which consisted of around one in seven (13.8 per cent) of the world population. Other major religions were Buddhism (7.1 per cent), Sikhism (0.4 per cent) and Judaism (0.2 per cent). Around one in eight people (11.2 per cent) belonged to other religions or are non-religious (9.4 per cent). In addition, there were 2.0 per cent avowed atheists. Of course, within each religious group there are likely to be those who are simply nominal members and also a variety of sub-groups. Below, we make observations on the attitudes to contraception and abortion of some major religious groups. However, few members of each group may follow official teaching. This is particularly true of Catholicism where few adherents follow the Pope in opposing artificial birth control or the Church's rigid attitudes to abortion.

Jewish Law

Although Jews make a small proportion of the world's population, their religion has greatly influenced the development of Christianity and Islam. The religion is sub-divided into three main groupings – Orthodox, Conservative and Reform – but within these groupings there are myriad subdivisions. In some ways the Orthodox are the most instructive in that they have a coherent, longstanding belief system. For example, adherents should not have sex until twelve days after the start of their menstrual period. Those with knowledge of the 'safe' period will see this as a recipe for fertility. Furthermore, when the time in the month is right then the man should have sex with his wife and sex is regarded as a *Mikvah* – a blessing. After women have a menstrual period they are regarded as unclean until they have had the ritual bath. Adherents are not allowed to work on the Sabbath, however, if they put tall masts around a designated area it is called an *Eruv* and it allows them to carry out a wider range of activities. As far as fertility control is concerned, Orthodox Jews are not supposed to use contraception. The religion does not recognize the foetus as being of equal status to the woman until the infant head is born. Once this has occurred 'the baby's life is considered equal to the mothers, and we may not choose one life over another' (Eisenberg 2007). However, in the womb the life of the foetus is subordinate to that of the mother and may be sacrificed:

> If there is a direct threat to the life of the mother by carrying the foetus to term or through the act of childbirth, in such circumstance, the baby is considered tantamount to 'rodef', a pursuer after the mother with the intent to kill her. (Eisenberg 2007)

According to Eisenberg, Judaism recognizes psychiatric as well as physical factors as potentially posing a threat to the life of the woman. Rabbi Waldenberg would allow an abortion of a foetus with deformity that would cause it to suffer in the first trimester and the termination of a foetus with a lethal, inherited defect such as Tay-Sachs disease up until the seventh month of gestation. The only reference to abortion in the Bible is in Exodus 21:22, where it says that if a man 'hurt a woman with child so that her fruit depart from her, and yet no mischief follow: he shall be surely punished according as the woman's husband will lay upon him'. So if the woman recovers it is seen as a minor event but if the woman dies then it would be a case of 'life for life'.

We shall see that in the Catholic and Muslim religions there has been a debate as to when life begins. The Bible says: 'God formed man of the dust of the ground and breathed into his nostrils the breath of life and man became a living soul' (Genesis 2:7). So from this it appears that life begins at birth and this ties in with the forgoing. However, the Bible suggests waiting later than birth. In Numbers 3:15 it is said that for a census you should only number a male child from the age of one month. Similarly, in Leviticus 27:6, it states that only children who have reached the age of one month should have a monetary value (Halperin 2007).

Christianity

The largest world religion is Christianity. Originally it was a religion opposed to rigid rules. Although Christ was Jewish, he often broke the religious laws that were imposed. For example, he should not have performed healing on the Sabbath because it was regarded as work. However, the Bible tells how he healed a man with a withered hand. Over the years the various churches and sects increasingly introduced rules especially in the area of fertility. Christianity divided at an early stage into many different groups. The main division was, however, between the Orthodox (Greek and Russian) and the Roman Catholic versions of Christianity. Both groups enjoined restrictions on the sexuality of the clergy. The Catholic Church taught that all priests should be celibate but the Greek Orthodox Church only asked this of its higher clergy such as bishops.

The Catholic Church and Abortion

Until 1869, apart from the three-year period 1588–91, the Church held to a theory derived from Aristotle that a soul did not enter the male until 40 days after conception nor the female until eighty days after conception. So abortion could be carried out up until this time. As sex could not be determined it would not be difficult to argue for abortion until 80 days or nearly three months. The *Catholic Encyclopaedia* published in 1914 explained this fact from Aristotle's proposal had allowed abortion at the beginning of pregnancy and commented: 'The authority of his great name and the want of definite knowledge to the contrary caused this theory to be generally accepted up to recent times'. (*Catholic Encyclopaedia* 1914). There is also evidence of an indulgent attitude towards birth control. A French bishop consulted the Pope regarding a problem he was having with young married men using withdrawal as a method of contraception. He also found it difficult to convince the husbands 'that he is to be considered in a condition of mortal sin unless he either lives chaste in marriage, or runs the risk of having an unlimited family' (Francome 1984). In its reply (8 June 1842) the Holy See took a very gentle approach to the problem. It said that priests should not interrogate the men and if the wife should report the fact they should 'deal with it in the most tender manner' (Francome 1984, p. 24).

Things changed in the Church and one of the problems was a belief stated clearly in the British Catholic newspaper *The Universe* (22 May 1936) that 'It is now, and always has been, the mind of the Church that unbaptized infants go to Hell'. Due to this belief during the period 1869 until around the 1950s the Catholic Church took a view that abortion should not even be allowed to save the life of the woman. In a book *Moral Problems for Catholic Nurses* which was published with papal approval and in its fifth edition in 1935, it was stated that men often had to die in wars and similarly:

> A parallel case is the situation of a woman in a difficult labour, when her life and that of her unborn child are in extreme danger. In this situation it is the mother's duty to die rather than to consent to the killing of her child … better that ten thousand mothers should die than one foetus is unjustly killed. (Finney 1935, p. 46)

One reason for the death of the woman is the attitude to pregnancies occurring in the Fallopian tubes (ectopic pregnancy). It is impossible for the pregnancy to go to full term and therefore it would seem logical that the tube should be removed. However, as the *Catholic Encyclopaedia* explains, the Church decided on 20 March 1902 that an abortion in this case was not lawful. Similarly in 1935 Finney asked 'If a surgeon, operating … discovers an ectopic foetus not yet viable, is it lawful for him to remove it'. He continued to say 'No it is not' (Finney 1935, p. 14).

In the years after the Second World War the Church changed its attitudes and its leaders seemed to forget its earlier position, so that in 1963 Britain's leading Catholic Layman, Norman St John Stevas, stated that the Catholic Church had never objected to an abortion for ectopic pregnancy (1963, p. 40). We have seen that the evidence does not support that statement. In fact, we shall see that in Chile, even in recent years, women have been forced to continue an ectopic pregnancy until it becomes life threatening. Furthermore in Ireland in October 2012, Savita Halappanavar died because she was denied treatment during pregnancy.

Some people like to call themselves 'pro-life'. However, sometimes when restrictive Catholic doctrine is written into law it acts against women becoming mothers. Strict Church teaching opposes artificial insemination by donor and in

2007, a Church-inspired restrictive law caused the closure of the Novum clinic in Warsaw. This had been providing *in vitro* fertilization and it led to Beata Skolimoska, who was fourteen weeks pregnant and waiting for a check up, to comment that she was a 'believer in the Catholic Church' but that she was 'very frustrated by the religious policy adopted by the Government. I wanted to try the clinic again for a second child.' However, reporters stated that it was the man who was the most anguished at the clinic and could not believe why people should deny him and his wife of the chance of having a baby (Perlez 2007).

Prenatal screening, with the option of abortion if the pregnancy becomes problematic, has allowed couples to try for a baby. For example, each child of couples who are carriers of Tay-Sachs disease has a 25 per cent chance of having a genetic abnormality that causes death by the age of five years old. With prenatal testing and the option of abortion, these couples can plan for a healthy family and avoid having a child who will inevitably die at an early age. Without the availability of prenatal testing and termination many such couples would choose not to have children.

Other Christian Groups

The Methodists were the religious group which was among the first to support contraception in Britain and then to support the liberalization of abortion. Lord Soper, its well-known life peer, was a vocal supporter and the Methodist Conference called for liberalization in 1966. The Church of England was more ambivalent about the change in the law. However, the Church Assembly Board of Social Responsibility passed a resolution to liberalize the law in 1965. Other groups to pass a resolution in favour of the Abortion Bill were the Congregationalists, the Church of Scotland, the Free Church Federal Council and the British Council of Churches (Francome 1984, p. 87).

In the US, conservative Baptist communities tend to oppose abortion and there was at one time the so called 'moral majority'. This was formed by Jerry Falwell in 1979. Richard Viquerie wrote in *The New Right* (1981), 'There are an estimated 85 million Americans, 50 million born again Protestants, 30 million morally Conservative Catholics, 3 million Mormons and 2 million Orthodox and Conservative Jews with whom to build a pro-family, Bible-believing coalition.' One of the weaknesses of this assessment is that it is not a majority but rather a third of the US population. Also, not all the morally conservative groups will line up to oppose abortion. The Seventh-Day Adventists, for example, take issue with the anti-abortionists. K.D. Paulson, writing on the group's position, commented that the Adventists refused to criticize abortion in the same way as other Christian Conservatives and opposed Christians trying to get governments to make it illegal. He commented that the ancient Egyptians condoned abortion and that one papyrus lists information as to how to induce one. He also argued that abortion did not come with legalization but that in the 1920s one quarter of pregnancies ended in a termination. He commented that making abortion illegal was ineffective and as an example drew attention to the fact that from 1948–1958, 32 people were accused of abortion in Massachusetts and not one was convicted. He was vitriolic about the violence against abortion clinics in the US and said it revealed 'the satanic spirit behind much of the so called "Pro-Life" movement (Paulson 2007).

Muslims

There is scope for wide variation in beliefs as the Koran does not mention abortion. The majority of orthodox Muslims in recent centuries permitted abortion until the end of four months due to a belief that the soul enters the foetus at this time. The Republic of Egypt produced a pamphlet entitled 'Islam's attitude toward family planning' in which it says:

> Jurists of the Shiite Zaidiva believe in the total permissibility of abortion before life is breathed into the foetus, no matter whether there is a justifiable excuse or not.

The Iranian Grand Ayatollah Y Saanei commented 'If there are serious problems God sometimes does not require his creatures to practise his law. So under some conditions – such as parent's poverty or over population – then abortion is allowed'. (*LA Times*, 29 December 2000).

Other Muslims take the view that 'abortion does not abruptly become prohibited at a certain stage, but becomes increasingly disfavoured as the foetus develops' (personal communication). This belief has allowed the development of manual vacuum aspiration in Muslim countries. It is this procedure which we shall see has reduced the number of unsafe operations in Bangladesh.

Other Religions

Hinduism is the oldest of the world's major religions. It originated in India and spread to Nepal and Southeast Asia. It is a tolerant religion and accepts that other belief systems such as Christianity or Islam have value. It has the belief that individuals should connect themselves to the Brahman or Godhead. This is the spiritual source of the tangible universe (Wright 2006, p. 494). They also believe in reincarnation with one's subsequent status being dependent on one's actions. The cycle of reincarnation is ended when one obtains liberation from the finite world through self discovery.

Buddhism was established by S. Gautama (563–483 BC) who was born into Hinduism. At the age of 29 he left his wife and young son to seek enlightenment. The Buddha means the enlightened one and the idea is that those who become enlightened pass into *nirvana* in which 'ideas and consciousness cease to be'.

There are about 350 million Buddhists in 92 countries (Wright 2006, p. 496). On abortion they believe the woman must make the decision herself (Childbirth by Choice 2007).

The Sikh religion was founded by Guru Nanak in the 16th century and advocates a search for eternal truth. It has around 19 million adherents worldwide and nearly all of them live or have originated from the Punjab region of India. The Sikhs believe that the women's right far outweighs the right of the embryo/foetus – it is not given the status of a human person (Childbirth by Choice 2007). The Jains are a breakaway group established in the 6th century AD and have a belief in the non-injury of living things and are vegans. The religion was established in India and currently has around five million adherents. There are a variety of other religions groups including Shintoism and the Bahai founded in Iran in 1844. As we have seen all of the major religions of the world are sub-divided into different groupings.

Medical Developments

One important development is that of manual vacuum aspiration (MVA). This makes use of a simple syringe with a plunger to generate the necessary pressure for uterine evacuation. The amount of negative pressure obtained by MVA is similar to that generated with a large expensive electrical pump. So it can be used in low-cost settings and after use can be sterilized or disinfected to be used again. (Grimes et al. 2006).

An important innovation is that of medical abortion. Marge Berer writes

> Medical abortion is the use of pills to cause a miscarriage. It represents a particularly important advance in abortion technology because it brings women's access to safe abortion closer to home … Medical abortion has been shown to be safe for over 15 years now, and as the word of its existence has spread, women all over the world have been using it, including in remote parts of developing countries. (2005, p. 6)

The WHO recommends the combined use of mifepristone and misoprostol as being better than either one alone. Misoprostol was first use as a drug to prevent and cure ulcers and it is relatively cheap and available (Grimes et al. 2006). Women take the mifepristone tablet by mouth, and the misoprostol tablets are inserted vaginally or taken by mouth. This vaginal insertion can be effected by the woman, her partner or the provider. Women having such an abortion 'do not need a hospital bed, in fact they don't need a bed at all' (Berer 2005, p. 8)

By 2005, more than 22 million women in China, one million in France and around three million in the rest of the world had had medical abortions and found it safe. In some areas of Norway it is now offered as the main abortion method and women must request otherwise if that is their choice. In Scotland in 2005 three in five (59 per cent) abortions were medical ones. In England and Wales it was below half this figure (24 per cent). Medical abortion has also grown in popularity in India. It is also suggested by observers that in areas of the world where there are restrictions on legal abortion, such as Africa, Latin America and some parts of Asia, misoprostol has been increasingly self-administered by women as an alternative to much less safe methods. Observers in Latin America in 2005 commented: 'Interest in the use of medical abortion has been growing during the past decade throughout Latin America using mainly misoprostol' (Lafaurie et al. 2005). Such self administration led to the drug being banned in Brazil, which we shall see only served to create a black market and drive up the price. Indeed observers suggest that the self administration of misoprostol during the period 2000–2005 led to a reduction in maternal deaths due to abortion in both Brazil and Peru and a review of death certificates in an urban area of Mexico found no deaths due to first trimester abortion 'perhaps in part because of the increasing use of medical methods (Lafaurie et al. 2005, p. 76). An in-depth study of 49 women who had medical abortions found that many women were happy with the lack of disruption to their lives. A 27-year-old government office administrator in Colombia said:

> The advantage is that you can go on normally with your life ... While I was going through this I went to work like always. I just had to be careful about the bleeding, just like when you have a heavy period .... Normal, it's totally normal, you just go on with your life as you normally would.

In this study the cramps were the most common side effect, reported by 46 of the 49 women. These were described as very strong by 17 women. Respondents pointed out that the most intense pain lasted two or three hours. However, in this study they were not following the WHO guidelines (Lafaurie et al. 2005, p. 79).

The Dutch group Women on Waves (WOW) has been one of those pressing for misoprostol (also known as Cytotec) to be used in countries with no legal abortion. There was a special International Day of Action on unsafe abortion on 28 September 2013 and WOW sent out an upbeat press release in support. It drew attention to the great profits on erectile drugs made by Pfizer and that they were going to give a proportion of their profits to helping provide Cytotec to women in poorer countries:

> Finally, men can take the leading role to improve women's health and protect their lives. From now on all men can turn their sexual pleasure into a life-saving experience. (WOW 2013)

Another development that has had some impact on safe abortions is the provision of contraceptive information to those who are in contact with the health services either to gain an abortion or to be treated for the after effects of an unsafe operation. Research in Zimbabwe found that when contraceptive services were provided it reduced the number of future unwanted pregnancies by 50 per cent (Grimes et al. 2006).

Structure of the Book

In this book I analyse the situation in all countries for which information is available and have populations over 10 million – this will cover around ninety per cent of the world's population. I have also included a number of smaller countries where there is special interest: for example, Israel as the only country with a majority of people of the Jewish religion and Ireland as a country with strong Catholic links and an anti-abortion statement written into the constitution. I use the United Nations classification of continents and consider countries in alphabetical order within each region. In considering each country the aim is to provide some basic facts about the country, followed by a discussion of contraception and abortion. One of the questions I have considered is whether there are any societies in the world which have been able to successfully convince its population to abstain from premarital sex, or alternatively, in countries whether where such attempts are made, contraception is not encouraged and abortion is largely illegal it leads rather to unsafe operations or women becoming sexual tourists. I draw conclusions from the findings in the final chapter.

Chapter 2
Europe

'The rhythm method was no good for young Czechs. They didn't want to have sex according to a calendar. They wanted to have sex when their parents weren't home'.

Radim Uzel

The population of Europe was estimated at 140 million in 1750. It grew to 401 million in 1900 which is almost a tripling in size. During the nineteenth century the population grew rapidly in all European countries except France, Spain and Ireland (Royal Commission on Population 1949, p. 7). In the period 1970–75 the average woman had 2.2 children. It fell to 1.6 in the period 1990–95 and to 1.4 from 1995–2000 (UN 2004, p. 29). Table 2.1 gives a country by country analysis of fertility.

Table 2.1 Average number of births in 2013

Eastern Europe							
Belarus	1.5	Bulgaria	1.4	Czech Rep.	1.3	Hungary	1.4
Moldova	1.6	Poland	1.3	Romania	1.3	Russia	1.6
Serbia	1.4	Slovaka	1.4	Ukraine	1.3		
Northern Europe							
Denmark	1.7	Estonia	1.5	Finland	1.7	Iceland	1.9
Ireland	2.1	Latvia	1.3	Lithuania	1.3	Norway	1.8
Sweden	1.7	UK	1.9				
Southern Europe							
Albania	1.5	Bosnia & Herze.	1.3	Croatia	1.4	Greece	1.4
Italy	1.4	Portugal	1.5	Slovenia	1.3	Spain	1.5
Western Europe							
Austria	1.4	Belgium	1.7	France (2011)	2.1	Germany	1.4
Liechtenstein	1.7	the Netherlands	1.8	Switzerland	1.5		

Source: CIA 2013. Selected pages p. 6 (Albania) to p. 766 (UK).

Table 2.1 shows the birth-rate is well below replacement level for European countries. There is also a general consistency with virtually all countries having rates between 1.3 and 1.9 children per woman. Only France and Ireland have over two children per woman. A large change has occurred in predominantly Catholic countries such as Italy, Spain and Portugal which were formerly known for their

Table 2.2 Maternal and infant mortality rates

	Maternal mortality per 100,000 2010	Infant mortality deaths in the first year 2013	Population millions July 2013
Eastern Europe			
Belarus	190	3.7	9.6
Bulgaria	11	15.6	7.0
Czech Republic	5	3.7	10.2
Hungary	21	5.2	9.9
Moldova	41	13.3	3.6
Poland	5	6.3	38.4
Romania	27	10.4	21.8
Russian Federation	34	7.2	142.5
Serbia	12	6.3	7.2
Slovakia	6 (2008)	6.4	5.5
Ukraine	32	8.2	44.6
Northern Europe			
Denmark	12	4.1	5.6
Estonia	2	6.8	1.3
Finland	5	3.4	5.3
Iceland	5	3.2	0.3
Ireland	6	3.8	4.8
Latvia	34	8.1	2.2
Lithuania	8	6.1	3.5
Norway	7	3.5	4.7
Sweden	4	2.7	9.1
United Kingdom	12	4.5	63.4

Source: CIA 2012, p. 67 (Belarus) to p. 766 (UK).

large family sizes. However, it is not only Catholic countries where the birth rate has declined. During the period 2005–9 Albania's rate was 2.2 and declined by seven children for every ten women by 2011 (CIA 2012, p. 6).

Within the generally low birth rates there have nevertheless been some increases. Both France and Ireland expanded their birth rates from 1.9 children in 2000–2005. Furthermore, a number of other countries increased their birth rate at least a little. In Greece, for example, the rate grew from 1.2 during 2000–5 to 1.4 in 2013.

The data for maternal and infant mortality rates are provided in Table 2.2. A note of caution: Stan Henshaw comments that maternal mortality and infant

Table 2.3 Maternal and infant mortality rates Southern and Western Europe

	Maternal mortality per 100,000 deaths 2010	Infant mortality deaths in the first year 2013 est.	Population size millions 2013
Southern Europe			
Albania	27	13.7	3.0
Bosnia and Herzegovina	8	6.0	3.9
Croatia	14 (2008)	6.0	4.5
Greece	3	4.9	10.8
Italy	4	3.3	61.5
Portugal	8	4.5	10.8
Slovenia	12	4.1	2.0
	6	3.4	47.4
Western Europe			
Austria	4	4.2	8.2
Belgium	8	4.2	10.4
France	8	3.3	66.0
Germany	7	3.5	81.1
the Netherlands	6	3.7	16.8
Switzerland	8	3.8	8.0

Source: CIA 2013, selected pages from p. 6 (Albania) to p. 700 (Switzerland).

mortality rates between countries may not always be meaningful. For example in recent years the maternal mortality rates in the US rose because of expanded efforts to locate deaths of pregnant women who died of other causes though possibly related to the pregnancy. On the question of infant mortality he states that what may be called a stillbirth in one society could be registered as an infant death in another (Personal communication). However, despite these provisos there are clearly differences between societies that indicate where improvements in health could be achieved.

The results for Eastern and Northern Europe show that the median rate of maternal mortality is that of 11 per 100,000 in Bulgaria. Belarus has a surprisingly high rate which is 17 times the median rate. Moldova, Latvia and the Russian Federation all have rates over three times the median. The Northern European data shows maternal mortality rates which are generally lower. The figure for Ireland is half that of the UK which is particularly surprising in that over the period Irish doctors did not always terminate a pregnancy if the woman's life was in danger. It is possible that some women whose lives were threatened moved to the UK. The rate for the UK at 12 per 100,000 is one of the highest in Northern

Europe and suggests that an improvement in care may be needed. The rates in Estonia, Finland, Iceland and Sweden are all below half the UK 2010 rate.

The infant mortality rates for Eastern and Northern Europe show the median rate to be that of the 6.1 for Lithuania. The highest rate is that of Bulgaria with Moldova second and Romania third highest. Sweden and Ireland were the two countries with the lowest rates.

The results for Table 2.3 show that for Southern and Western Europe the median maternal mortality rate is 8 per 100,000 births. The highest rate is Albania with 27 deaths per 100,000 maternities. This contrasts markedly with the lowest figure of only three for Greece. In Western Europe the rates are generally low with the highest being the figure of eight in three countries.

The infant mortality rates for Southern and Western Europe show the median rate to be 4.2 for Austria and Belgium. Again, Albania had the highest rate with three times the rate for the median of the group. The lowest results were the 3.3 deaths per 1,000 live births in France and Italy.

Europe: A Divided Continent

There are still fairly strong differences in family patterns between Eastern and Western Europe. In the past Western European marriage differed from Eastern Europe in at least two main ways. The first was that Western Europe had a high average age of marriage, and secondly it had a high proportion of people who never married. It is a unique feature of North Western European civilization and lacks a satisfactory explanation (Stone 1977). In 1900 the Western European pattern of marriage extended broadly to the West of a line running from St Petersburg to Trieste. If we consider a selection of countries from the West of Europe there is a pattern. So Austria, Germany, Great Britain, Holland, Italy and Sweden each had at least sixty per cent of its women single in the age group 20–24 years and at least one in ten of its women were single in the age group 45–49 years. In contrast, if we consider Hungary, Romania, Bulgaria, Serbia and Greece they had earlier marriages and so in each case the majority of the 20–24 age group were married. In Serbia for example 84 per cent of women 20–24 were married. Furthermore, in Serbia only one per cent of women were single by the age group 45–49 years, in Bulgaria it was two per cent, Romania three per cent and Hungary and Greece four per cent. With young marriages there were other differences such as the marriages often being arranged by the parents (Hajnal 1965). Some differences in marriage patterns still remained in Europe this century. For example, in Eastern Europe younger women 15–29 provide 83 per cent of the births while in Western Europe it was only 63 per cent (UN 2004 34). The UN reported in 2004 that there were several European countries where the average age of marriage for women was over thirty. These were Finland, France, Iceland, Ireland, Norway and Sweden.

The WHO reports that Eastern European women who wanted a small family have had little access to modern contraceptives. Consequently and by default, abortion became the major means of limiting fertility in many Eastern European states. The WHO states that although abortion is legal in these countries, many procedures are carried out under insanitary conditions or by poorly trained providers. Consequently, the complication of unsafe abortions recently accounted for 25–30 per cent of maternal deaths in Russia and an estimated 50 per cent in Albania (Population Information Program 2007).

Although Eastern European family patterns are still very different from Western European ones there is an opportunity to move away from the reliance on abortion by improving contraceptive services. In May 2013 an article argued that abortion rights were under attack in former 'iron curtain' countries due to pressure from the Catholic and orthodox churches and the low birth rates. Wanda Norwicka, a reproductive rights activist who from 2011 was deputy speaker of Parliament in Poland commented: 'The gap between the eastern part of Europe is growing, especially when the issue has to do with abortion'. Further to the Polish proscriptions she drew attention to attempted restrictions in Ukraine, Lithuania and Croatia. 'Many policy makers in the region think there will be more children if they restrict abortion' (AFP 2013).

We now consider analysis of the situation in larger European countries.

Austria

The population was estimated at 8.2 million in 2013 and its life expectancy at birth was 80.0 years. Its religion is 74 per cent Catholic, 12 per cent none, five per cent Protestant, four per cent Muslim and five per cent, other. In 2011 the birth rate was 8.7 per 1,000 and death rate was 10.3. Immigration however, meant that the population was increasing slightly. Its infant mortality rate was 4.3 per 1,000 births in 2011. In the 1930s the country had the lowest birthrate in the world and in the 1980s it had the third lowest birthrate after Germany and Italy (Perner 2007). In 2011 the average woman had 1.4 children (CIA 2012, p. 45). The capital city, Vienna, had a population of 1.7 million in 2009 (CIA 2012, p. 45). One observer commented that since the 1970s there has been a great increase in the defections from the Catholic Church 'especially because of the sexual morals of the Church which are no longer accepted by many of its believers' (Perner 2007).

At the Hague Forum of 1999 the Austrian government's view was that it was not called upon to directly influence reproductive behaviour. Rather that suitable family policy is to remove, or at least to minimize, those structural obstacles which stand in the way of individuals in their decision to have children. In this respect it outlined a number of measures.

- To improve childcare facilities and especially help women with children below school age.

- To provide single parents with 18 months off work to care for a child. For couples it was to be an extra six months to divide between the couple in order to encourage fathers to play a more active role.
- To carry out job audits on the helpfulness to families and provide Government awards to companies which had family-friendly policies.
- To provide family counselling for those who requiring it in 305 different centres.
- To improve access to family planning to help reduce the abortion rate.
- To ensure that family planning was not a population tool but rather a means of extending people's choices
- To make artificial reproduction 'routine' so that more women could benefit.

More recent data reveals that in Austria the higher the job qualifications for the woman the lower the percentage of unwanted pregnancies. By 2007 the country had over 200 publicly supported family planning and partnership counselling centres. As in other countries there was some movement away from the contraceptive pill in the 1970s with scares about its possible side effects. Women increased usage of the IUD and sterilization. However, still around 42 per cent of fertile women 15–44 were using the contraceptive pill in 2005 (Perner 2007).

The Austrian abortion law came into operation under a socialist Government on 1 January 1975. It was opposed by the Catholic Church which sponsored a 'national petition for the protection of human life'. It was signed by 895,665 people, which was almost 18 per cent of eligible voters. Austria does not keep records of the number of abortions. The country has allowed *in vitro* fertilization since 1992 (Perner 2007).

Belgium

The population was estimated at 10.4 million and life expectancy at birth was 79.8 years in 2013. Its religion is 75 per cent Catholic. In the year 2013 the birth rate was 10.0 per 1,000 and the death rate slightly higher at 10.6. This gives a slight decrease in population. The capital city is Brussels with a population of 1.9 million (CIA 2013, p. 70)

Belgium made abortion illegal in 1810 and it was legalized in 1990 in part by an extraordinary manoeuvre. The king told the Prime Minister that he could not sign a liberalizing measure into law as he was a Catholic. There was the potential for a constitutional crisis. It was solved by the Government declaring the king unable to rule and it assumed his authority and enacted the law. The next day the Parliament voted to reinstate the king and he was only out of power for 44 hours. The Vatican said the king had made 'a noble and courageous choice'. The Church was opposed to the law and one critic talked of the fact that 'thousands of unborn babies are being aborted in Belgium by wicked mothers (Ngambi 2005). In fact the Belgium abortion rate is relatively low and in 2009 only 12 per cent of pregnancies were terminated which is well below other comparable societies.

There was an unusual case brought before Bruges Criminal Court when two doctors and a nurse were charged that they did not wait the requisite six days between first appointment and operation when carrying out an abortion on a 14-year-old girl. The girl herself was 18 at the time of the case which she had brought herself. A supporter of the doctors said in court that in 25 per cent of cases the six days waiting time is not adhered to 'due to the woman's urgency and distress' (Genethique 2005).

Czech Republic

The population was estimated at 10.2 million and its life expectancy at birth was 77.6 years in 2013. One in ten is of the Catholic faith and under one per cent Protestant. The vast majority are unaffiliated or unspecified (CIA 2012, p. 195). In the year 2013 the birth rate was 8.6 per 1,000 and the death rate 11.0. The capital city, Prague, has a population of 1.3 million (2011 estimate). Czechoslovakia under Alexander Dubcek denounced Stalin and abolished censorship. However, the brief 'Prague Spring' ended in August 1968 when the Warsaw Pact forces invaded. The Slovaks and Czechs separated on 1 January 1993 and democratic elections occurred in 1996.

The Czech Republic has tended to use abortion instead of contraception. Some western observers have commented that this suited some leaders as it meant they could control fertility in a way which they could not if women had access to up to date contraception. The abortion law was liberalized in 1956 and in 1957 extended to non-health reasons. However, between 1956–86 women had to seek the permission of abortion commissions. This was readily given, however, and led to a high number of abortions (Baranik 2006). In the 1980s there were around 116,000 abortions a year and little use of modern methods of contraception. Alena Kralikova commented 'Communist leaders sought total control over citizens'. The contraceptive pill was available but less than 10 per cent of fertile women used it. The population tended to use withdrawal or the rhythm method either or which were not very reliable. Radim Uzel commented 'the rhythm method was no good for young Czechs. They didn't want to have sex according to a calendar. They wanted to have sex when their parents weren't home' (Francome and Vekemans 2007, p. 18). The increase in modern methods of contraception during the 1980s led to the number of abortions dropping to 58,000. In 2004 the use of the pill had increased to two in five fertile women and the number of abortions reduced to 27,574 which is less than a quarter of the level in the 1980s (Francome and Vekemans 2007, p. 18).

France

The population was estimated at 66.0 million in 2013 and its life expectancy at birth was 81.6 years (2011 est.). Religion is 83–88 per cent Catholic, two per cent Protestant one per cent Jewish and 5–10 per cent Muslim. In the year 2012 the birth rate was 13 per 1,000 and the death rate 9 per 1,000. This gives a rate of natural increase of 0.4 per cent. The capital city, Paris has a population of 10.4 million (CIA 2012, p. 258).

French law made abortion illegal in 1810 and the country had a long history of unsafe abortion (Francome 1984). Tardieu claimed in 1868 that it had increased into a 'veritable industry' and by the end of the century several observers noted the rise in hospital admissions for abortion (Potts et al. 1977, p. 161). In 1907 a French physician, M Tissier, stated that magistrates took a light view of abortion and that upper class women had no shame in stating that they had had one. In the same report a Dr Blondel talked of 'sundry English women, both married and unmarried, who had crossed the Channel simply to have an abortion brought on' (Francome 1984, pp. 33–4). Other evidence on this issue is provided by a Mrs Burgwin who visited France around 1913 and told the Birth Rate Commission that over and over again, doctors had told her that rich English women went to Paris for abortions (1917, p. 220). One had said 'We have got 50,000 criminal abortions taking place in Paris in a year and we find numerous English women resort to that city to be relieved of their pregnancy'. This trade continued at least until the 1930s (Francome 1984, p. 34).

In the aftermath of the First World War, the French Government was concerned that its population needed to be increased. In 1920 it introduced a law which even banned contraception. So France was in a strange position where abortion was provided for foreign women but birth control was illegal. It seems that in France there were attempts to reduce the number of illegal operations and in 1950 2,885 people were sentenced for abortion. By 1969 the number was reduced to 471 and the sentences reduced (*The Times* 15 November 1974). One case which brought the issue to prominence was the Bobigny affair, which concerned a girl, aged 17 who had obtained an abortion following rape. Her trial took place in November 1972 at Bobigny near Paris. She was acquitted; her mother received a fine and the abortionist a suspended sentence (Francome 1984, p. 138).

We have seen in previous works that in both Britain and the US activists wishing to change the law had to decide whether to go for the right to choose in the early part of pregnancy or whether to go for more limited change and allow abortion for rape, incest, foetal abnormality or for social reasons. In France there was an attempt at such a limited bill in 1970 introduced by a Gaullist deputy but when this failed the advocates of free abortion decided to demand repeal by an aggressive campaign. A total of 343 women signed a manifesto published in the left-wing magazine *Le Nouvel Observateur* stating that they had had an abortion and calling for repeal. The list included famous actresses and authors such as Catherine Deneuve, Jeanne Moreau and Simone de Beauvoir and none could be prosecuted because the offences were out of time (*The Times* 15 November 1974). Public opinion was in favour of change and the *Catholic Herald* reported that almost 60 per cent of the population was in favour of abortion on demand in the first ten weeks of pregnancy (27 December 1974). Simone Veil, the Minister responsible for the preparation of the Bill, claimed that 300,000 French women had abortions each year despite its illegality. This estimate seems high in the light of subsequent experience. However, the problem of law enforcement was encapsulated by the Minister of the Interior who said that it would have been necessary to send more than fifteen million women to prison in the previous fifty years (*The Times* 15 November 1974).

The legalizing of abortion on request until the tenth week of pregnancy occurred on 17 January 1975. In 1979 the abortion rate was half the rate in the US. The law was initially on five years trial. It was somewhat slow to come into operation but then increasing availability led to the number of women travelling to England for abortion dropping rapidly (Francome 1984, p. 140). In 1974 a total of 36,541 French women were recorded as having abortions in England and Wales. Two years later the number was down to 4,459 and would have been lower but for the short gestation period allowed by French law (Francome 1986, p. 57).

In 2009 there were 209,314 abortions on French women and 793,420 live births. This meant just over one in five (20.9 per cent) pregnancies ended in abortion. At the beginning of 2013 it was announced that French women were to receive free contraception and abortion from 1 April. The aim was in part to promote contraception in order to reduce the abortion rate. There were some who opposed the change and thought some women take abortion too lightly, however, Plank commented 'Abortions are not like half price Easter chocolates. Women don't run out and get them because they are on sale. They get them because they need them' (2013).

Germany

The population was estimated at 81.1 million in 2013 and life expectancy at birth 80.3 years. Its religion is one third (34 per cent) Protestant and one third (34 per cent) Catholic. In addition there are four per cent Muslims and three in ten (28 per cent) are unaffiliated. In the year 2013 the birth rate was 8.4 per 1,000 and the death rate 11.2. The capital city is Berlin with a population of 3.4 million in 2009 (CIA 2012, p. 279).

The German abortion law was based on the Prussian Penal Code of 1851 which was adopted by the German Reich in 1871 (Kommers 1977). We saw that in April 1971 famous French women publicized their abortions. Inspired by this less than two months later (2 June), 24 well-known actresses, journalists and singers had their photographs on the front page of *Stern* news magazine. All had signed a declaration saying that they had broken German law. These were part of a wider protest where 374 women had concurred with their admission. The youngest was 14 years old and the oldest 77. The supporters of liberal abortion used these admissions to argue that the law was unworkable. One of the organizers, Ingrid Huebner, was quoted as saying 'If all the women who have had an abortion had the courage to take out a summons against themselves the law would be swamped by a flood of 5 million trials'. In theory, under German law, state attorneys have no choice but to prosecute even in cases where a person is self-accused. Actress Romy Schneider, despite having a warrant threatening to prosecute her, flew to Bonn to a party given by the Chancellor Willy Brandt. This act contravened the terms of the warrant and gave further publicity to the cause (*New York Times* 24 June 1971).

The situation in Germany became very acrimonious with the women's movement arguing that their lives were being controlled by religious doctrines to which they did not subscribe. Churches were daubed with the slogan 'Ban 218' which referred to the relevant clause. On Easter Sunday 1974, the Primate had his service at Munich Cathedral interrupted by a tape-recorded attack on him being released from a confessional booth.

Availability of abortions in other countries led to German women travelling elsewhere. In 1970 3,621 women went to Britain for abortion and the figures quadrupled to 17,531 in 1972. Even more went to Holland and it was estimated that in 1975 a total of 61,000 German women travelled there for abortions (Francome 1986, p. 57).

Legalization in East Germany in 1972 meant that its women had rights to control their fertility which were not available in West Germany. Parliament passed a law providing for abortion on request up to twelve weeks in 1974 but it was referred to the Constitutional Court. One year later this Court ruled the law out despite the fact that a poll showed three in five Germans supported it (Francome 1984, p. 142) However, revised legislation in 1976 allowed access to abortion and by 1979 the number of women travelling to Holland had halved from the situation five years earlier (Francome 1984, p. 143). The unification of Germany led to a great reduction in birth rates in former East German areas. In Brandenburg the number of births fell to a third – from 38,000 in 1989 to 12,000 in 1993. In fact in 1994 the regional Government began paying women $650 if they had a child (Lautmann and Starke 2005).

Greece

The population was estimated at 10.8 million in 2013 and life expectancy from birth was 80.2 years. Its religion is 98 per cent Greek Orthodox and 1.3 per cent Muslim. In the year 2013 the birth rate was 8.9 per 1,000 and death rate was 10.9. Despite this, however, the population showed a very slight increase due to immigration. The capital city is Athens with a population of 3.3 million (CIA 2013, p. 289).

We have seen that Western Europe has traditionally differed from Eastern Europe in that it has had a much higher age of marriage and a much greater percentage of women who never married. Greece comes between the two systems and shares some of the characteristics of each. However, the average age of marriage has increased from 22.3 years in the 1980s to 25.9 in 1998. The average

age of the first child also increased from 23.3 in the 1980s to 28.6 in 1998. Evidence of the continuing respect for marriage in Greece comes from the fact that in 1998 only 3.8 per cent of births occurred outside marriage (Ionnidi-Kapolou 2004). One commentator states on the position of Greek women:

> Traditionally there has always been strict control of women's sexuality, especially in the countryside, with the men of the family responsible for keeping an eye on their daughters and sisters so they do not have sexual relations before or outside marriage. (Ionnidi-Kapolou 2004)

The country developed its family planning clinics in 1980 when the Minister of Health established it in the public sector by law. Ten family planning centres were established. However, progress has been slow and Greece has had one of the lowest rates of use of modern contraceptives in Western Europe. They have also concentrated on male methods so in 1997 41 per cent of couples used condoms and a further 31 per cent used withdrawal. This is presumably one of the reasons that the country's abortion rate has been one of the highest in Europe. In the 1970s it was estimated that annually there were 300,000 illegal abortions. Women's organizations became active on the issue and on contraception which was illegal in Greece until 1980.

In 1983 the Greek National Health System was formed and included information and education on family planning matters amongst its targets. There was a ratio of 1:1 abortions and births (Ionnidi-Kapolou 2004).

In 1986 abortion on request was introduced within the first 12 weeks of conception. In cases of rape, incest or seduction of a minor the limit was 19 weeks and for serious foetal abnormality it was 24 weeks (UN 2013, accessed 23 December).

Halkias reports that in the mid-1990s the number of abortions were estimated at 300,000–400,000 which given the population size would mean that Greece had the highest or second highest rate in Europe. He reported that it then dropped to 200,000–300,000 later in the decade (2005). The UN reports that the number of abortions did not markedly increase after legalization as abortion was already widely reported. It continued to say that it was difficult to estimate the actual number of abortions. They could be done speedily outside hospitals in a doctor's private surgery and if so would not be recorded. Consequently we do not have accurate data on the numbers (UN 2013).

Ireland (not including Northern Ireland)

'Abortion is absolutely the most emotive, divisive issue in Irish society' said an Irish journalist and there does not appear to be a solution at the moment (Hallan 2012).

The population of the country was estimated at 4.8 million in 2013 and its life expectancy at birth was 80.4 years. Its religion is nearly nine out of ten (87 per cent) Catholic and five per cent other Christian. In the year 2013 the birth rate was

15.5 per 1,000 and the death rate 6.4 per 1,000. The capital city is Dublin with a population of 1.1 million (2009).

Ireland wrote strict Catholic doctrine into its law on contraception. The Courts decided that Irish people could legally use contraception but that it was also legal for the Government to ban people from obtaining them. In 1971 a group of feminists travelled from Belfast in the north and brought condoms to Dublin. The pressure paid off and contraception was legalized in 1980. However, a prescription was needed until 1985 (McDonald 2012). Since that time contraception has spread so that from 2005–2010 modern methods were used by 65 per cent of women of childbearing age which is higher than the world average.

The Irish abortion law is based on the British Offences against the Person Act 1861). Public Opinion on social issues has historically been very different to the rest of Europe and the United States. For example a survey in 1973/4 found that 54 per cent of Irish people agreed with the statement 'Divorce should never be allowed'. And seven out of ten stated that sex before marriage is 'always wrong'. It also found that 91 per cent of Catholics went to mass each week. On modern methods of contraception one third saw them as 'always wrong'. The difference between other countries can be seen from the fact that in a 1980 Gallup Poll in Britain, the US and Ireland asked a similar question on abortion. In the US and Ireland the question was 'Do you think abortion should be legal under any circumstances, only under certain circumstances or illegal in all circumstances?' In Britain the phrase 'legal under any circumstances' was substituted by 'legal on demand', but otherwise the question was identical. The results showed a great difference between Ireland and the other two countries. Whereas four out of five of the Irish thought abortion should be 'illegal in all circumstances', only one in five Americans and one in eight British residents shared their view (Francome 1984, p. 215). Catholics in Northern Ireland were more liberal than those in the south and 35 per cent would allow abortion in some circumstances.

We have seen that in other countries of the world when abortion is illegal there is a great problem with unsafe operations. However, in Ireland since 1968 women have been able to travel to England. In 1970, 261 Irish women had abortions in Britain. This number increased to 3,603 in 1981 (Francome 1984, p. 215). There then followed a steadier increase to 4,200 in 1991 and to 4,900 in 1996; then in 1999 there were 6,200 rising to a high of 6,400 in the year 2,000. By this year most other countries had legalized abortion and women from these countries did not find it necessary to travel to Britain. Consequently, more than four out of five (80.5 per cent) of the 9,800 non-resident women having abortions in Britain were from Ireland (both north and south). There has been a move for Irish women to obtain their abortions in Holland and Belgium where they are cheaper (personal communication).

The abortion law in Ireland is out of line with other main European countries and in 2009 the European Court ruled that Ireland's total ban on abortion was in breach of women's human rights. Its relevance came into focus when an Indian Hindu dentist Savita Halappanavar died in a Galway Hospital on 31 October 2012 after being refused a life-saving abortion and spending days in agony. She was told 'this is a Catholic country'. Her husband, Praveen, commented 'How can you let a young woman go to save a baby who will die anyway' (Holland 2012).

Public opinion in Ireland is moving away from the Catholic Church. We have seen in 1980 four out of five Irish citizens said that abortion should be illegal in all circumstances. Change has been such that in May 2013 a poll found that seven out of ten (71 per cent) of Irish citizens agreed with an abortion where a woman had been raped and almost seven out of ten (69 per cent) agreed that abortion should be available for 'the long term risk to the health of the mother.' So Irish opinion has changed (O'Hanlon 2013). The Halappanavar death meant there was strong pressure for a change in the law. This resulted in a minor liberalization of the abortion law in the summer of 2013. The first abortion under the law was reportedly carried out at the Hollie Street Maternity Hospital in Dublin which was one of twenty five in the republic authorized to carry out terminations under the new law. However, there was some confusion about the date the new law came into operation (McDonald 2012).

Italy

The population was estimated at 61.5 million in 2013 and its life expectancy from birth was 82.0 years. Its religion is four out of five Catholic and approaching one in five atheists. In the year 2013 the birth-rate was 8.9 per 1,000 and the death rate 10.0 per 1,000. The capital city is Rome with a population of 3.4 million (2009).

Contraception was opposed by the Fascists and in 1930 a law introduced one year detention for anyone promoting it. The law was kept after the Second World War and continued despite the fact that in the 1950s over half of poor families had five or more children (DeMarchi and DeMarchi ND). The DeMarchis were a husband and wife team who in 1956 opened a centre for contraception. It was illegal, but their first client was a police officer who had been sent to investigate. He had four children and was happy to find out how to avoid more. He left with the name of a doctor saying that he was going to report back that everything was under control. Maria DeMarchi visited the poor area of Rome called Borgate and reported that the poor realized the rich had fewer children and wanted to know why. One woman – Filomena – had five children and eight previous abortions and said that she had a great need for contraception. In an odd development a representative of the Vatican placed himself outside the DeMarchis' home and began taking photos of those visiting. Photographs were then given to local priests who warned their flock about Maria DeMarchi: 'What she will give you is dangerous to your health and can give you cancer'. The DeMarchis kept up their agitation for many years. After the Pope published *Humanae Vitae*, Maria DeMarchi wrote *Inumanea Vite* [Inhuman Lives]. In 1964 the pill began to be used in Italy. This development was not welcomed by the Pope. Maria DeMarchi helped organize a group of women to disrupt the Easter message with large banners saying: 'Yes to the pill, No to the population bomb.' There was worldwide publicity including the front page of the *New York Times*. Despite having the support of public opinion it was not until 1970 that the courts overthrew the 1930 ban on information about contraception (DeMarchi and DeMarchi).

It seems that abortion was common in Italy even before the First World War. In a large trial in 1904 eight licensed midwives were convicted of what the *British Medical Journal* (BMJ) called 'abortion mongering' (*BMJ* 28 May 1904). In 1975 the WHO estimated there were 1.5 million abortions a year, the Italian authorities estimated 800,000 and the woman's movement 3 million a year (*Economist* 25 January 1975). A poll in 1976 showed that over three in five (63 per cent) of Italians wanted a new law.

The abortion law in Italy was slightly liberalized by a Supreme Court decision in 1976. However, it was changed to give women abortion on request on 28 May 1978. The impulse to change the law derived much of its impetus from the developments in France. *The Times* stated: 'France's decision to legalize abortion has left many Italians with a feeling of bitter isolation … all Italy's northern neighbours have now give their women the right to terminate pregnancies under decent and controlled conditions' (6 December 1974).

The campaign in Italy was very different from that in France and Britain where the pro-choice organizations tried to keep a more respectable image and argue, for example, that abortion would protect the family. In contrast, Italian feminist groups began confrontational tactics. The Centro Informazione Sterilizzazione e Aborto (CISA) aimed to help women directly and make the country face up to the issue. It introduced suction abortion to Italy and accompanied women to inexpensive practitioners, or, if their pregnancy had passed three months, to London. It was headed by Adele Faccio, a 55-year-old single woman who bore a son at the age of 36. She was speaking in Paris when she learned she was to be arrested and gained maximum publicity by announcing she would give herself up at a large abortion rally in Rome. She returned to Italy with the help of borrowed documents and a wig to force the arrest to take place in front of the press, television and hundreds of supporters. The *Times* commented: 'The episode has the desired effect of turning Adele Faccio into a heroine and martyr and making the embarrassed carabinieri officer appear the stooge of an obtuse regime bent on imposing its crude fascist laws' (15 April 1976).

One of the crucial issues during the debate was the relationship between Church and State. This problem had become accentuated with the 'Seveso' case when an explosion led to women being exposed to a chemical known to cause foetal malformation. The Christian Democrats allowed 38 women to have abortions, which was a decision that caused a rift with the Vatican (*Catholic Herald* 20 August 1976, *Universe* 7 July 1978).

In 1978 the law was changed to allow abortion in the first trimester for medical, economic, social, family or psychological reasons or if there was a defect in the foetus. In 1979, the first full year after the Act 188,000 legal abortions occurred at the expense of the state (Francome 1984, p. 146). The country had to decide whether or not to overthrow the law in a referendum. The Catholic Church played an active role and the *Observer* commented 'The Pope has virtually entered the hustings' (3 May 1981). The people defeated the 'pro-life' amendments with 67.9 per cent of people opposed to it. Even before the voting Joan Lewis in Rome for the *Catholic Herald* predicted the final result:

> There is a silent majority in this predominantly Catholic country which admits that abortion is here to stay, however heart rending and agonizing the problem. The more vocal of this majority argue that it would be better to search deeper and find the causes of this 'social plaque' as they call it. They say that abrogating the current law would not eliminate abortions and indeed, could encourage clandestine abortions, which have a high mortality rate'. (Francome 1984, p. 146)

After the law was passed the number of abortions grew to a recorded peak of 228,974 which was 27.1 per cent of all pregnancies. By 2010 the number of abortions recorded had almost halved to 115,517 which suggests that the contraceptive services have improved greatly (Johnston 2013c).

The Netherlands

The population was estimated at 16.8 million in 2013 and life expectancy at birth was 81.0 years. The religion is 30 per cent Catholic, 20 per cent Protestant, 42 per cent unaffiliated and six per cent Muslim. In the year 2013 the birth rate was 10.9 per 1,000 and the death rate 8.5 per 1,000. The capital city is Amsterdam with a population of 1.0 million (CIA, p. 517).

The great difference between developments in Holland and those in other countries is that the big increase in quasi-legal abortion preceded any liberalization of the law. In 1911 the law was changed so that abortion was considered to be a crime against public morality (Ketting and Schnabel 1980). From this time onwards there were abortions only on 'medical grounds' and in the 1950s an estimated 10,000–15,000 illegal abortions a year (Treffers 1965, p. 58).

Although the Dutch were amongst the first pioneers of contraception in the nineteenth century, it appears that progress has been slow. One strong belief reported was that a birth control mentality was a major cause of induced abortion and this was to be discouraged. However, with the introduction of the pill in 1964 it became accepted that contraception could prevent abortion, and in a small country such as Holland use of the pill spread rapidly. In 1969 the ban on birth control advertising was lifted and by 1971 the cost of the female-orientated contraceptive methods were covered by the country's public health insurance and therefore free of charge. By 1977, 41 per cent of Dutch women aged 15–44 were on the pill – by far the highest usage in the world at that time. In the period 2005–2010, 69 per cent of women 15–49 used contraception.

The change in attitude to contraception had led to different attitudes about abortion. For in cases where contraception had failed physicians felt responsible and women began to assert their right to control their own fertility. In 1966 an eminent Dutch law professor Ch. J. Enschede concluded that the concept of what was 'medical' had become much broader amongst physicians and that this should apply to abortion as well. He concluded that doctors were well within their rights under the law if they carried out abortions on a wide variety of social grounds, such as if the woman were single or had completed her family. The statement seems to have taken the medical profession by surprise. However, in the following year it was approved in Parliament by the secretary of Justice, and it became accepted that any abortion carried out in proper conditions by a doctor was legal (de Bruijn, 1979, p. 192, Ketting and Schnabel 1980). In the late 1960s there was, however, a shortage of capacity and in 1970 816 Dutch women had their abortions in England. However, the setting up of specialist clinics from 1971 abrogated the need for women to travel and in 1973 only 101 Dutch women received abortions in England (Francome 1984, p. 136). Indeed, foreign women began to travel to Holland for their operations. Although the abortion rate for resident women was low – only around 5.2 abortions per 1,000 women 15–45 years, the influx of foreigners was estimated by Stimezo –the Dutch National Abortion Federation – to be as high as 61,000 from Germany, 12,000 from Belgium and 9,000 from France in 1975 (Ketting and Schnabel 1980).

Despite the low abortion rate and presence of legal abortion it was controversial to introduce a bill to regularize the situation. As I have documented more fully elsewhere, there were a total of eight bills in eleven years, before in 1981 a bill allowed abortion on request up to twenty weeks in specially licensed clinics. There was a restriction of a five day 'meditation' period between the request and the operation (Francome 1984, p. 137).

Abortion is free to Dutch women living in Holland.

A news programme in 2004 reported that the Government was abandoning the policy of free contraception for all. Some observers argued that the Netherlands had amongst the lowest abortion rate in the world but that this change might lead to an increase. This was especially true because immigrant groups had 60 per cent more abortions even amongst those born in Holland. This was in part because immigrants were caught between two cultures – the conservative ones of their parents and the more liberal ones of Dutch society (Roxburgh 2004). In the event the number of abortions was 28.8 thousand in 2003 and rose to 33.0 thousand in 205 before dropping to 26.7 thousand in 2010.

Of course this reduction might have been even greater if free contraception had continued. In 2010 there were 183,866 births. This means that excluding stillbirths and miscarriages the percentage of pregnancies ending in abortion was one in eight (12.7 per cent) which is relatively low as we see from the data in other countries.

Norway

The population was estimated at 4.7 million in 2013 and life expectancy at birth was 80.4 years. Religion is 86 per cent Evangelical Lutheran, three per cent other Protestant and one per cent Catholic. In the year 2013 the birth rate was 10.8 per 1,000 and the death rate 9.2 per 1,000. The rate of maternal mortality fell from around 500 deaths per 100,000 births in 1880 to 10 per 100,000 in 1979 and 4.6 per 100,000 in the 1990s which is one of the lowest rates in the world. The capital city is Oslo with a population of nearly 900,000 (CIA 2012, p. 544).

The first clinic offering advice related to sexuality and childbearing was opened in Oslo and others followed. Contraceptive advice was limited at first. However, it gradually expanded and by the 1960s when modern contraceptives became increasingly available, there was already a tradition of family planning. In 1999 the Government made a decision to provide free condoms to all young people under the age of twenty. These were introduced to help reduce the abortion rate and as a strategy to reduce the incidence of HIV and sexually transmitted infections. Furthermore, from 2002, Parliament decided that women under the age of 20 were to receive free contraceptive pills (Austveg and Sundby 2005). The policies led to the Norwegians having 88.4 per cent of women aged 15–44 using contraception which is the highest percentage recorded in the world (WHO 2012).

The Norwegian abortion law of 1687 did not distinguish between abortion and infanticide and punished both with the death penalty. Capital punishment was replaced by hard labour and prison in 1842. The Penal Code of 1902, which remained in place until 1964 did allow abortions if they were justified by a doctor. However, a number of illegal abortions resulted in maternal deaths. These rose steadily at the beginning of the twentieth century and then doubled during the decade 1920–30. During the period 1930–40 the deaths rose only slightly but they were high during the years 1940–5, although local observers say some of this might be due to better reporting (Austveg and Sundby 2005, p. 25). In post-war years illegal abortion deaths began to fall quite rapidly until they were much lower by the early 1950s (Austveg and Sundby 2005). In 1964 a law came into force calling for hospital medical committees to decide all individual cases. A study in 1973 documented social and geographical differences in the decision of doctors and medical committees as to whether legal abortion should be provided. The modern law came into operation in 1979. It allows 'abortion on demand' in the first 12 weeks of pregnancy and by a decision of a medical committee over twelve weeks (Austveg and Sundby 2005, p. 25).

When legalization occurred some felt that the rate would rise. However, that did not. In 1980 the abortion rate was 16.3 per thousand aged 15–45 It fell to 14.5 by 2008 (Johnston 2013d). Abortion rates amongst adolescents (under 20 years) fell by about a fifth between 1982 and 2002 despite the fact that the reported age of first intercourse was reduced. Clearly this is due to improvement in contraception.

Norway was one of the pioneers in the introduction of *in vitro* fertilization treatment in public hospitals.

Poland

The population was estimated at 38.4 million in 2013 and its life expectancy at birth was 76.5 years. Its religion is 90 per cent Catholic (about 75 per cent practising). In 1920 the birth rate was 37.6 per 1,000 population and declined to 22.3 in 1960 (Francome 1984, p. 130). In the year 2013 the birth rate was 9.9 per 1,000 which is below a third of its 1920 level. The death rate was 10.3 per 1,000. The capital city is Warsaw with a population of 1.7 million (2009 estimate) (CIA 2012).

In Poland a 1932 law allowed abortion for the sake of the woman's health and for rape and incest. Abortion was legalized on request in 1955 and this led to Swedish women visiting the country for terminations. In 1965 the *New York Times* (14 February) reported that Swedish law stated that it was illegal to do abroad what it was illegal to do in Sweden and so 20 women were threatened with prosecution. This resulted in great opposition and a revision of the Swedish law. In 1978 Poland had 145,600 abortions recorded, which is a rate of 18.3 per 1,000 women aged 15–44, although this figure is recognized as being incomplete (Francome 1984, p. 129). A woman named Maria told me of her experience:

> In 1987 I was just splitting up from my husband of sixteen years. We had never used contraception and only had one child. When we broke up I had a brief affair with a policeman. He was very high up not one who was on the streets. He was married and I was very surprised when I became pregnant. I did not feel I had any choice but to have an abortion. He paid for me to go to a private clinic and the abortion was very painful. The cost was equal to a month's pay. (Interview 3 April 2007)

Since the country has been independent of Communist rule the law has been very controversial. First, abortion was restricted in 1993 and there was some concern about illegal abortion which was a factor in the law being offered on wider grounds in October 1996. It figured heavily in the election of the following year which led to it being restricted once again. This current law allows abortion for the woman's health or life, for foetal abnormality or for such crimes as rape or incest. However, there is further pressure from the right to make abortion illegal even for rape. The Prime Minister Jaroslaw Kaczynski rejected this call from the League of Polish Families to provide the 'right to life from the moment of conception'. He was quoted as saying 'Can a sovereign and democratic state oblige a woman who has been raped to have a baby. In my opinion it cannot.' Such a restriction would not have the support of public opinion as only one in five (20 per cent) wanted stricter abortion laws (Easton 2007).

It is estimated that there are 200,000 illegal abortions a year and the illegal sector is said to be 'thriving' (Moore 2003). Many women also travel to the Czech Republic where abortion is legal and the Swedes have stated that they should help Polish women who want abortions to repay the favour for earlier periods where Poland provided abortion for Swedish women as we have discussed (Francome 2004). However, Polish women have died because of the recourse to unsafe abortions. For example, in March 2005 Karina Kozak underwent an illegal abortion in the private apartment of a gynaecologist. After the procedure she haemorrhaged and was taken by ambulance to a hospital where she died. Less than two months later a 25-year-old pregnant woman became ill during pregnancy and the medical profession did not carry out the correct procedure. The doctor said he was going to perform an endoscopy, which carries the risk of miscarriage, but decided against it 'My conscience won't let me do it'. The woman died and Professor Rydzewska said that if the endoscopy had been performed it would have identified the source of infection and the problem could have been solved (Nowicka 2005, p. 162). So we can see that the re-introduction of illegal abortion to Poland is creating a difficult situation.

The Dutch group 'Women on Waves' visited the country in 2005. The group moored their boat in Wladyslawowo but planned to go to international waters in order to provide women, who were up to six weeks pregnant, with RU 486. Its leader Dr Rebecca Gomperts commented 'What I can tell you is that we've had more than 200 telephone calls from the public. Women are desperate here. You cannot imagine how a woman feels when she has an unwanted pregnancy. She doesn't want a child and she feels so lonely. It is very sad and moving when you talk to these women.' (Moore 2007) Other women said that the presence of the boat had led to an opening of debate and discussion. For example 20-year-old Olga set out her experience a year earlier. She was about to take exams and commented:

> I was not ready to have a baby. I answered an ad in a newspaper and found a doctor. I had to pay a lot of money for the abortion. I think it is a good idea that Women on Waves came to Poland. More women feel confident about discussing abortion now' (Moore 2003)

A case to the European court has thrown the law in Poland into some disarray. Alicja Tysiac became pregnant with her third child. She went to see three specialists who all said that continuing the pregnancy was likely to cause deterioration in her vision. However, as they felt the potential deterioration was not certain they refused to sign for her to have an abortion. She continued with the pregnancy and her eyesight deteriorated to such a degree that she could only see up to five feet away. She took the Polish Government to the European Court of Human Rights and in March 2007 was awarded €25,000 compensation. At the press conference following the decision she commented:

> Every woman should decide herself whether she wants to have the baby or not and the Government should not mix into that at all … . In Poland there is no work, people have nowhere to live and it is hard to see your own child hungry or to deny it things.

In addition to these comments Wanda Nowicka alleged 'Thousands of women are denied abortions that they are legally entitled to in Poland every year' (Easton 2007, Hennesy and Smyth 2007).

We saw in the introduction that a Polish clinic providing *in vitro* fertilization was ordered to close in 2007 because it was said to breach the abortion law. One in six Polish couples are estimated to suffer from infertility problems (Perlez 2007).

In 2011 anti-abortion activists obtained over 500,000 signatures to have abortion banned altogether. The bill was narrowly defeated by 191 votes to 186 in the August. In September 2013 the Bill came up for vote again. Marta Szostak wrote for the International Campaign 'Today was a big day in Poland' when the bill to ban abortion for foetal malformation was voted down. This came at the time when there were meetings worldwide to campaign against unsafe abortion. Irina Otmakhova pointed out that in addition to the success in Poland over fifty other countries were taking action.

Portugal

The population was estimated at 10.8 million in 2013 and its life expectancy at birth was 78.9 years. Its religion is 85 per cent Catholic, however, only one third are regular churchgoers. In the year 2013 the birth rate was 9.6 per 1,000 and the death rate 10.9 per 1,000. The capital city is Lisbon with a population of 2.8 million in 2009 (CIA 2012, p. 584). The setting up of democracy in 1974 led to women's rights being a crucial issue. The new Constitution introduced in 1975 recognized the right to a new 'conscious parenthood'. Despite its Catholic heritage Portugal increased its contraceptive usage until during the period 2005–2010 nearly nine out of ten (87 per cent) of women aged 15–49 and in relationships used contraception which was the second highest level in the world.

In contrast, abortion remained a crime for longer. In 1976 the Family Planning Association was founded and the abortion issue was brought to prominence by a film called, ironically 'Abortion is not a crime'. It showed an abortion by use of a Karman's cannula and bicycle pump, and made it reasonably easy to see how to carry one out. The programme also included a discussion in a dimly-lit room with a group of women who explained why they had had abortions. The journalist, who wrote the script, Mario Palla, was charged in 1979 with 'assault on public morals' and incitement to crime. Palla's position on the issue was clear 'To legalize abortion is a real, concrete way to make women more free. People who are against the liberalization of women are against abortion' (Francome 1984, p. 213).

A bill was passed in 1984 which allowed abortion in the first 12 weeks of pregnancy for the woman's health and for rape until 16 weeks. There was pressure to further change the law and in 1998 a referendum asked the following question: 'Do you agree with decriminalization of abortion when requested by women's demand up to 10 weeks of pregnancy and performed in an authorized clinic'? The response rate was low with only 32 per cent of the respondents voting. A bare 50.1 per cent voted 'No' (CNN 2007). This, of course, did not end abortion and in the period 2007 around 40,000 abortions were estimated to have occurred each year. The richer women could go to Spain and clinics were built just over the border in relatively easy reach of Portuguese women. Others were carried out locally by *partieras* –'capable women'. These were part of a long tradition. As long ago as 1979 one of the activists Madelena Barbosa was quoted as saying: 'Some of the midwives are really quite good, they use proper medical instruments and operate in sterile conditions'(Francome 1984, p. 214). There were several high profile prosecutions on the grounds of illegal abortion. One such was of J.A. Pinto, a social worker, who said that every week he had to face women who wanted illegal abortions. He was freed on appeal but others were sent to prison. A new referendum took place on 11 February 2007 and it had the support of the socialist Prime Minister who was quoted as saying 'We have to end this plight of backstreet abortions. It makes Portugal a backward place' (Catalinotti 2007). In a referendum 60 per cent of the respondents were in support of a new law. However, although the turnout was increased to 44 per cent, it did not reach the 50 per cent required for the decisions to be mandatory.

In 1985 Spain liberalized abortion which meant that Portuguese women had the opportunity to travel there for safe operations. An abortion centre was set up in the Spanish border city of Badajoz and by 2007 it was carrying out 4,000 abortions a year, nearly all of them on Portuguese women. At this time a new referendum was being anticipated and in the event three in five (59 per cent) Portuguese voted for a liberal law. It gave abortion on request until 10 weeks, although there was a three-day mandatory waiting period so women had a period of reflection.

Romania

The population was estimated at 21.8 million in 2013 and its life expectancy at birth was 74.5 years. Its religion is nearly nine out of ten (87 per cent) Eastern Orthodox. In 2013 the birth rate was 9.4 per 1,000 and the death rate slightly higher at 11.9 per 1,000. The capital city is Bucharest with a population of 1.9 million (2009 est.).

Contraceptive use increased from over half (57 per cent) married and cohabiting women in 1990 to two thirds (65 per cent) in the year 2,000. However, only one in three (31 per cent) of women were using modern methods of contraception (UN 2004, p. 57).

Abortion was first legalized in September 1957 following legal changes in the Soviet Union. Romania provides a good example of what can happen to women's health if abortion is prohibited. In 1966 the Government was concerned about declining fertility and population so placed stringent restrictions on the liberal abortion act. Decree 770 stated that abortion would only be allowed for women under the following conditions:

- They had given birth to and raised four or more children, or were over 40 years of age.
- They suffered from, or had a spouse who suffered from a severe hereditary disease which might be transmitted.
- They had severe physical, psychological or sensory disabilities that would prevent them from caring for the newborn.
- Their life was threatened or the pregnancy was the result of rape or incest.

Until this point the number of deaths from abortion had been falling. They halved from 130 in 1961 to 64 in 1965. However, they then almost tripled to 170 in 1967 and increased by over five times to 364 in 1971. This rise in abortion deaths was clearly related to the growth in unsafe operations after the increased criminalization. Over the same period the birthrate shows the effect of the law. It was 17.5 per 1,000 population in 1961 and steadily fell together with the abortion deaths to 14.6 per 1,000 in 1965. Then, with the 1966 abortion restrictions, the birthrate almost doubled to 27.4 in 1967. However, as the number of illegal operations began to rise, the birthrate steadily fell and by 1971 it was 19.5 per 1,000 which is lower by almost a third from the peak (Francome 1976, p. 392).

The restrictive abortion law in Romania lasted for 24 years until December 1989 when the dictator Nicolae Ceauşescu was ousted and the new Government provided abortion on request. Observers commented:

> Although abortion became much safer, quality of care was severely limited by the heavy demand for services. In the early 1990s the disastrous effects of Ceausescu's extreme pro-natalist anti-family planning policies on women's sexual and reproductive lives were documented. (Johnson et al. 2004, p. 184)

Once the law changed the deaths from abortion declined. In 1989 the maternal mortality was 170 deaths per 100,000 live births and 87 per cent of all maternal deaths were abortion related. The rate more than halved to 84 per 100,000 in 1990 and then to 53 per 100,000 in 1993. This decline was due almost entirely to the decrease in abortion related mortality from 148 per 100,000 live births in 1989 to under a quarter –34 per 100,000–in 1993. By 2002 abortion related mortality was down to 9 per 100,000 (Johnston et al. 2004, p. 186). The exceptionally low rates of contraception led to the country having possibly the highest abortion rate in the world from 1990–2. Teams assessing abortion interviewed a woman in the Roma community who stated she performed 24 abortions on herself with a pen and had no complications. Of course on some occasions she may not have been pregnant (Johnston et al. 2004, p. 189). The rate at this time was 182 abortions per 1,000 women of reproductive age which is around thirty times the rate of some other Western countries such as Germany, Holland and Belgium. It is instructive to consider the changes in births and abortion in Romania

Table 2.4 Romania: percentage of pregnancies ending in abortion (excluding foetal deaths and miscarriage

	Births	Abortions	Births plus abortions	Percentage terminated
1990	314,746	992,265	1,307,011	76%
2000	234,521	257,865	492,386	52%
2010	212,199	101,920	314,119	32%

Source: Johnston (2013L).

Table 2.4 shows that in 1990, the first full year of the liberal law, the number of abortions was nearly one million and that three-quarters of pregnancies ended in termination. Ten years later in 2000 the number of abortions decreased to below a third of their former level. Just over half of pregnancies terminated. A further 10 years later and the number of abortions had declined by more than half and less than a third of pregnancies ended in abortion. In fact in the 21 years between 1990–2010, the number of abortions declined in every single year. This is as contraception has been substituted for abortion (Johnston et al. 2013l,). Henshaw comments on the figures:

> I believe the number of abortions declines sharply but the later figures exclude increasingly numbers performed in private physicians' offices, so we do not know how much. (Email 2 December 2013)

In Romania it is local general practitioners rather than gynaecologists who provide contraceptive counselling and by the end of 2003, 2,300 out of approximately 15,000 family doctors had been trained together with 1,750 nurses (Johnson 2004). Furthermore, the Ministry of Health implemented a programme that provides free contraceptives to poor and disadvantaged women. So further reductions in the number of abortions may be expected.

Russian Federation

The Soviet Union under the leadership of Mikhail Gorbachev introduced *Glasnost* (openness) and Perestroika (restructuring) in an attempt to modernize Communism.

His initiatives released forces which led to the formation of Russia and fourteen other independent republics by the end of 1991 (CIA 2012, p. 598).

By 2013, its population was estimated at 142.5 million and life expectancy at birth was 69.9 years. Its religion is 15–20 per cent practising Russian Orthodox and 10–15 per cent Muslims. There is a large group of non-practising believers and non-believers. In part this was because during the Communist years the dominant ideology was atheism. In the year 2013 the birth rate was 12.1 per 1,000 and the death rate 14.0 per 1,000. The capital is Moscow which had a population of 10.5 million in 2009 (CIA 2012, p. 598).

It was in the Soviet Union that abortion was first legalized in modern times and it strongly affected the debate in Britain and the US. As early as 1914 the most eminent society of physicians had called for all laws to be removed. In 1920 the Soviet Government faced with a high birth rate and a large number of unsafe abortions, passed a law legalizing the operation. It provided that abortions would be performed free of charge in hospitals.

The Soviet law had two main effects on the debate elsewhere. First, it was a prime example in showing that change was possible and radical groups were able to point to it as an example of what could be accomplished. Secondly, and this was probably more important, it revised the estimates of the safety of the operation. Until that time it had been believed that abortion was a very unsafe procedure. The Soviet Authorities drew comparisons with Germany where in 1924 four per cent of abortions were estimated to have resulted in death. In contrast, the Moscow death rate was less than one tenth of one per cent (Francome 1984, p. 63). The Soviets publicized their results and in 1929 sent a delegate to the First Congress of the World League for Sexual Reform in London. The figures suggested that abortion mortality and morbidity in the country had decreased 'almost to vanishing point'; British doctors took a great interest and on a number of occasions visited the country to observe the procedure. One such doctor was L. Haden Guest, who reported in *The Lancet* (5 December 1931) that in a Russian series of 40,000 abortions there were only two deaths. The US-based Dr F.J. Taussig paid a visit to the Soviet Union in 1930 and devoted a whole chapter of his influential book to the subject of legal abortion in the country (Taussig 1936, Francome 1984, p. 63).

In 1936 the Soviet Union repealed its law. The *New York Times* reported strong opposition from women who felt they would be condemned to being childbearing machines, commenting that the abortion law had not prevented the creation of happy, devoted and even conventional families. It argued that the change in the law was 'the first step toward putting the Soviet Union squarely into a population race with Germany and Italy (*New York Times* 7 March 1937). The change in the law was accompanied by promises of large premiums for every child after the seventh and there was also a crackdown on illegal abortion. In one case, 18 women were sentenced to between one and ten years in prison. The restrictive Soviet law continued to allow abortion if pregnancy threatened

Table 2.5 Abortions and births in Russia

	No. live births	No. abortions	Pregnancies (ab + births)	% abortions
1960	2,782,353	4,373,042	7,155,395	61%
1990	1,988,858	4,103,425	6,092,283	67%
2000	1,247,490	2,138,750	3,386,240	55%
2008	1,713,947	1,385,600	3,099,547	45%

Source: Johnston (2013k). Number of pregnancies excluding miscarriages.

the woman's health or if there was a likelihood of inherited disease (Francome, 1984, p. 63). The programme was initially effective and official estimates told of a tripling of the birthrate in Moscow in the first year (Francome 1984, p. 64).

The Soviet Union legalized abortion again in 1956 and the law became fully operational in 1958. It was legal on request up until 12 weeks and up to 20 weeks on a variety of social grounds. Russia was part of the Soviet Union in until 1991 and had a very high rate of abortion as can be seen from Table 2.5.

Table 2.5 shows that in 1960 there were over four million abortions and that three in five pregnancies were terminated. By 1990 the number of births had declined substantially but the number of abortions remained over four million and two in three pregnancies ended in abortion. In 1992 the Government began to subsidize contraception and during the 1990s the number of abortions declined. In 2000 they were down to 2.1 million. In fact during the period 1988–2001 the percentage of women using modern contraception increased by 74 per cent (Deschner and Cohen 2003, Johnston 2013k). This century the rate has continued to fall and in 2008 the number was down to under 1.4 million and the percentage of pregnancies ending in abortion was down to below half (45 per cent). WHO advises that during the period 2005–2010 almost four out of five (79.5 per cent) women in relationships used contraception. If this figure is correct we would expect the abortion rate to drop dramatically (WHO 2012).

With the resurgence of the Russian Orthodox Church and concerns with declining population there had been pressure to reduce the number of abortions by legal means and in 2003 the Government restricted the social grounds for abortion after 12 weeks gestation. The right to choose remained in the first 12 weeks. This was a relatively small change but nevertheless was opposed by Dr Yuri Bloshansky, who had been Moscow's chief gynaecologist for over 40 years. He commented 'I remember vividly the women dying, forced to go anywhere, going to swindlers operating in septic conditions' (Myers 2003).

Overall, it seems that Russia is gradually using contraception to a greater degree with there being a diminished reliance on abortion

Spain

The population was estimated at 47.4 million in 2013 and its life expectancy at birth was 81.4 years. Its religion is 94 per cent Catholic. However, local observers comment that church attendance is dwindling and less than 20 per cent go to mass regularly (Adler 2004, da Cunha e Tavora 2007). In the year 2013 the birth rate was 10.1 per 1,000 and the death rate 9.0 per 1,000. The number of births has increased from just under 1.1 per woman in 2000 to 1.5 in 2011(Western 2006A). The capital city is Madrid with a population of 5.8 million (2009) (CIA 2012, p. 676).

Contraceptive use increased from seven out of ten (70 per cent) married and cohabiting women in 1990 to 66 per cent during the period 2005–2010 (UN 2004, p. 57, World Bank 2012). At this level it is a little above the world average.

One of the first liberalizations of the abortion law in Western Europe was that in Catalonia, which in 1936 allowed abortion for foetal deformity, rape or 'sentimental' reasons in the first three months of pregnancy (Anderson 1980). The movement to the right under the rule of General Franco in the late 1930s led to abortion, birth control and divorce being made illegal. After Franco died a new constitution was set up which paved the way for birth control to be legalized in 1978 and divorce in 1981. In 1974 the Spanish Council of Scientific Investigations came to the conclusion that the abortion law was inadequate and should be revised. The setting up of a democratic system led to the parties dividing with the left wing groups such as the socialists being more in favour than the right wing groups (Anderson 1980). However, the major pressure for change came from the women's movement.

There were many court cases: in 1975 there were 151, and it was reported in the British women's magazine *Spare Rib* that a woman had received 10 years imprisonment (Francome 1984, p. 212). It was, however, the twice-suspended trial of 11 women in Bilbao which most galvanized opinion. Nine of the women had undergone abortions and almost all of them already had several children. The tenth person was the abortionist and the eleventh her daughter who had assisted. The trial began in October 1979. As in France and Italy, one of the most effective protests was from well-known women who stated they had had abortions. In Spain 4,300 women including a respected dramatic actress, the Eurovision Song contest winner, and a former Miss Spain signed a statement which in part pointed out 'Spanish justice is condemning women because they do not have the £250 which it costs to go to England for an abortion' (*Guardian* 25 October 1979). This protest brought great publicity to the trial and when it concluded in March 1982, ten of the eleven women were cleared. The abortionist, Julia Garcia, was found guilty but was recommended for an immediate pardon.

Many women began to seek legal terminations in Britain. The first record of Spanish terminations in the UK was in 1972 when 730 were completed. The number rose to 2,900 in 1974, reached 14,100 by 1978 and peaked at 22,000 in 1983. In January 1983 the newly-elected Socialist government published plans to liberalize the law in cases of rape, foetal deformity and risk to the life of the woman (*Daily Telegraph* 28 January 1983). The Spanish law was changed in 1985 and allowed abortion in some cases such as where the foetus is damaged, to avoid physical or mental harm to the woman or where rape or incest had been reported to the police. If these conditions were met Spanish Social Security would pay 75 per cent of the costs (Fuchs 2005). With this change in the law, the number of women travelling abroad began to fall; in the year of the 1985 Act, 17,700 women had abortions abroad. The number fell to 5,900 in 1987 and continued to fall to only 32 in the year 2,000 (Johnston 2013m).

The number of recorded abortions in Spain increased from 49,000 in 1995 to 85,000 in 2004 and 111,000 in 2010. This rise may have been in large part due to a decline in illegal abortion but there were those who took the view that the number of abortions could be reduced. Pilar Triguero of CEAPA, a national federation of 12,500 parent teachers associations asserted:

> We have to get rid of the taboos about sex education. The state funded schools tiptoe around the subject and they do not have an established curriculum. What is taught depends on the discretion of each teacher (Fuchs 2005)

There were also those who expressed concern that Spanish society did not support family life enough. For example Margarita Delgado, a demographer said that many women waited for a permanent job until they decided to start a family. Furthermore, she commented that Spanish businesses worked late hours which made it difficult for women to juggle jobs and children. She added that state support for families in Spain was one of the lowest in the European Union (Fuchs 2005).

When the socialist Government of Rodriguez came to power in 2004 it adopted a policy of reform on social issues and clashed repeatedly with the Catholic Church. It legalized gay marriage, eased divorce laws, and dropped religious education from the national curriculum (Govan 2009). A liberalized abortion law came into effect on 5 July 2010 and gave women the right to choose in the first 14 weeks of pregnancy. The number of abortions more than doubled from 54,000 in 1998 to 118,000 in 2011. Its abortion rate was still relatively low compared to some other countries (12.4/ 1,000 15–44 years). In the run up to the election the conservative People's Party stated its intention was 'to reinforce protection of the right to life'. It gained power and announced in Parliament in January 2012 that it was going to restrict abortions for minors. Later the Justice minister – Alberto Gallardon – said they wanted to return to the 1985 law but without allowing an abortion for foetal deformity. However, an article in June 2013 drew attention to political divisions which were leading the Government to be hesitant about putting the clock back (Parry 2013). Henshaw comments on the number of abortions:

> After 2010 a large proportion of recent abortions have been for immigrant women from Central and South America. This group accounts for part or all of the increase in abortions. (Email, 2 December 2013)

In 2014 there was a debate regarding restrictions of Spanish law. It is not clear for what purpose, but it will meet great resistance.

Sweden

The population was estimated at 9.1 million and its life expectancy at birth was 81.3 years in 2013. Its religion is 87 per cent Lutheran. In the year 2013 the birth rate was 10.3 per 1,000 and the death rate was 10.2 per 1,000. The capital city is Stockholm with a population of 1.3 million.

In the seventeenth century Sweden had made abortion punishable by death. However, in 1864 it reduced the punishment to six years in prison (Linner 1968). Sweden liberalized its law in 1921 but the restrictions meant that illegal abortion still continued and during the 1930s it was the cause of around 70 deaths each year. A Royal Commission was set up in 1934 and resulting legislation which went into operation on 1 January 1939. It allowed abortion if childbirth would entail serious danger to the life or health of the woman, if she were pregnant following rape or incest or under 15 years of age. It also allowed abortion in cases where the women were legally insane or if serious physical or mental handicap might result (Linner 1968, p. 76). In 1946 a further indication was added. This was to allow abortion if there were reasons to assume that childbirth and care would seriously undermine the woman's physical and psychic strength with reference to her living conditions and other special circumstances. In 1956 the Swedes made sexual education compulsory. The drug thalidomide gave great prominence to the abortion issue. It was first marketed for morning sickness in 1957 and was by 1962 known to be responsible for deformed children. The drug was not accepted in the US but a US journalist called Sherri Finkbine took the drug in England. When she could not get a legal abortion in the US, amid great publicity she flew to Sweden for her operation.

Although Swedish law was more liberal than others it was still very bureaucratic. In the period 1963–4 the patients at one hospital had an average of 26 days investigation and spent an average of 10 days in hospital (Potts et al. 1977). Abortion was more easily available in Poland and in the winter of 1964–5, 20 Swedish women were threatened with prosecution. Swedish law said that it was illegal to do abroad what it was illegal to do in Sweden (*New York Times* 14 February 1965). The predictable furore led to the prosecution being dropped and an eight-member commission to review the law which recommended in 1971 that abortion should be removed from the penal code, although abortions by lay persons should be illegal. In 1973 the law in Sweden was changed to allow abortion on request in the first 18 weeks of pregnancy. Between 12 and 18 weeks there must, however, be a discussion with a social worker (Francome 1984, pp. 132–4). In the 1990s the Swedish birth rate was higher than virtually all the countries in Western Europe. This has been linked to the introduction of 15 months of parental leave and a doubling in the number of day centres.

Table 2.6 Abortions and births in Sweden

	Births	Abortions	Abortions + Births	% Abortions
1990	123,938	37,489	161,427	23.2%
2000	90,441	30,680	121,121	25.3%
2010	115,641	37,698	153,339	24.6%
2011	111,770	37,750	149,520	25.2%

Source: Johnston (2013p)

One observer suggested that if other countries wished to increase their birth-rate they should provide parents with the time and resources to raise their children well (Arthur 1999). The Swedish abortion rate in the period 1998–2004 was just over 20 per thousand women aged 15–44, which we have seen is twice as high as countries such as Holland or Switzerland. It is interesting to consider the numbers of births and abortions in Table 2.6

Table 2.6 shows that the number of births fell by over a quarter between 1990 and 2,000 but have since risen. The percentage of pregnancies ending in abortion has been relatively consistently at around a quarter.

The Swedish law gave indigenous women the right to choose and in 2005 a Government commissioned report said the residential requirement should be waved. This was followed by an announcement on 16 January 2007. It was quickly picked up by Poland who suggested that Polish women would be able to get safe legal abortions in the country (Szczech 2007).

Ukraine

The country had a brief period of independence between 1917–20 but was then forced to face Soviet rule and two famines (1921–22 and 1932–33) during which over eight million died. In the Second World War the German and Soviet armies led to a further seven to eight million deaths (CIA 2012, p. 757).

It obtained its independence from the USSR in 1991 when its population was estimated at 44.8 million. In 2013 its life expectancy at birth was 68.9 years. In 2012 the birth rate was 9.5 per 1,000 and the death rate 15.8 per 1,000. So the population has been declining. The capital city is Kiev with a population of 2.8 million (2009 est.). The religious background is 92 per cent Eastern Orthodox although divided into different groupings. There are two per cent Roman Catholic two per cent Protestant with a few Jewish and other Christian groups (CIA 2012, p. 758). The Country had an extreme financial crisis in 1991–2. Inflation rose from four per cent in 1990 to 85 per cent in 1991. Part of the financial problems of the society were due to the nuclear accident in Chernobyl (CIA 2012, p. 758).

Table 2.7 Abortion and births in Ukraine

	Live Births	Abortions	Percentage pregancies aborted*
1990	657,202	1,019,038	60.8%
2000	385,126	434,223	53.0%
2005	426,086	263,590	38.2%
2010	497,689	176,774	26.2%

*Not including miscarriages
Source: Johnston (2013e)

Like the other countries of the former USSR the country has had a tradition of relatively low contraception and high abortion rates and significant figures can be seen in Table 2.7.

The figures show that in 1990, three in five pregnancies were aborted and that there were over a million abortions. Ten years later both the number of births and abortions were markedly reduced. However, from that period the numbers of births and abortions moved in different directions. The number of births rose by over 100,000 per year. In contrast, in every single year from 1999–2010 there was a decline in the proportion of pregnancies aborted.

These changes were in part due to a few initiatives by the Government. For example in January 2003 a new policy on the family was introduced. This made the legal rights of couples just living together much the same as those who were married. It aimed to increase financial support for women in the hope that this would reduce the number of abortions occurring for financial reasons. Furthermore in 2006 the Reproductive Health of the Nation was launched. This innovation aimed to provide better information on contraception for women. The data for 2005–2010 indicates that two thirds (67 per cent) of women in a relationship used contraception which is above the world average (World Bank 2013).

Despite these facts, in April 2012 the Nationalist Government brought forward draft legislation that proposed to restrict abortion and fine parents for not having children. Abortion would only be allowed in certain cases such as if the prospective father died, there was a genetic disability or pregnancy for an under-16. Andriy Shevchuk said the change would help to boost the flagging birthrate. In contrast, feminist groups said it would lead to illegal abortion. On 17 April 2012 they had a topless protest in a Cathedral and other acts of opposition. So it remains to be seen what if any restrictions will be imposed (White 2012).

United Kingdom

Great Britain consists of England, Scotland and Wales. The addition of Northern Ireland is called the UK. The population was estimated at 63.4 million in 2013 and its life expectancy at birth was 80.3 years. Its religion is 72 per cent Christian (Anglican, Catholic, other Christian groups). Almost one in four (23 per cent) are unspecified or have no religion There are about three per cent Muslim, nearly one per cent of both Sikhs and Hindus and 0.6 per cent Jews. In the year 2013 the birth rate was 12.3 per 1,000 and the death rate 9.3 per 1,000. The capital city is London with a population of 8.6 million (2009 est.) (CIA 2012, p. 766).

The early debate on contraception was rooted in the ideas of Thomas Malthus and his theory that there was a natural tendency for population size to outstrip food supply. He proposed that poor people should engage in self-restraint in order to restrict their family size. The neo-Malthusian movement altered his doctrine by suggesting people should use contraception rather than restraint. Two of its members Charles Bradlaugh and Annie Besant republished a booklet about contraception called *The Fruits of Philosophy*, and were brought to trial. The Solicitor General argued that the real aim of the book was 'to suggest to people that they might enjoy the pleasures of sexual intercourse with or without marriage and yet avoid offspring' (*The Times* 19 June 1876). The Lord Chief Justice took a similar line and said that up to now unlawful intercourse led to the birth of offspring and so the removal of this restraint 'may remove one of the restraints on vice and one of the safeguards on morality (Francome 1984, p. 36). They were initially found guilty but freed on appeal and the great publicity led sales of the book to increase from around 1,000 a year before the trial to 125,000 copies between March and June 1877. From that time onwards condoms were sold.

Until the First World War the neo-Malthusians were the only group promoting contraception. The socialists might have been expected to be supportive. However, Marx called the work of Malthus a 'shameless plagiarism' and socialists said the way to eradicate poverty was by a wholesale change in the social order (Francome 1984, p. 43). After the First World War there was a significant change. In 1921, Lord Dawson, the King's physician, called for the Church of England to accept birth control and in 1930 he was successful in getting a change. In 1921 Marie Stopes opened the country's first birth control clinic. In the 1920s the Catholic opposition to contraception became more active under an organization called the League for National Life. Sutherland, its leader said the propaganda for birth control had spread through the country 'until it reached the invisible and invincible frontiers of the Catholic church'. In spite of the opposition's efforts the Government became supportive and in 1931 the Ministry of Health first permitted advice on birth control to be given in antenatal clinics'. Contraception has been available free via the NHS since 1974. It is easily available via family planning clinics or GPs. However, GPs do not usually supply condoms (Bury and Ngo 2009). In the period 2005–2010, 84 per cent of women in relationships used contraception which is the fourth highest in the world (World Bank 2012).

Abortion was made illegal in 1803 in large part to protect the health of women. There were two other Acts before the 1861 Offences Against the Person Act which still stands today (although heavily amended). This act said that a person should not 'unlawfully' end a pregnancy. This implies there were lawful conditions for example to save the woman's life. However, it was ambivalent. The first call for legal abortion was that of Stella Browne in 1915. She argued for legalization on three grounds. First, she said that contraception was not perfect so it needed a backup, secondly that young people were not well educated and ignorance should not be punished and thirdly, that it left people open to blackmail (Francome 1984, p. 64). Shortly after her article was published reports came in of French women raped and made pregnant by German soldiers. The *BMJ* noted that there was sympathy that such women should be able to obtain abortions (20 March 1915). The Abortion Law Reform Association (ALRA) was set up in 1936 and had its first success in 1938 when a girl of 14 was raped and became pregnant. The doctor concerned, Aleck Bourne, was told 'she was with two girl friends, who ran off and left her, and she was held down by five men and twice assaulted' He was then asked 'whether someone of your standing were prepared to risk a *cause celebre* and undertake the operation in hospital'. Bourne agreed 'I have done this before and have not the slightest hesitation in doing it again' (Francome 1984, p. 70). He was tried under the 1861 Act and acquitted and from that time onwards abortion was considered legal for rape. In fact the judge made the point that a doctor who, for religious reasons, did not perform an abortion to save a woman's life: 'would be in great peril of being brought before this court on a charge of manslaughter for negligence' (Francome 1984, p. 70).

There were several bills to change the law. The Liberal MP David Steel was third in the ballot. His bill passed on 27 October 1967 and came into operation six months later. One debate towards the end of the discussions was on the degree of risk to the pregnant woman necessary for a legal abortion. The Lord Chief Justice, proposed 'abortion should be legal if the risk to life or the risk of injury to health was greater by continuing the pregnancy rather than terminating it. The Home Office said the wording was not a profound change. However, Norman St John Stevas, the prominent Catholic MP, said that if abortion was as safe as the reformers claimed then abortion would always be legal (Francome 1984, p. 99). He proved to be right.

In the early days of the Act the number abortions grew and the number of deaths from unsafe abortions rapidly fell. In 1980 the abortion rate was 12.8 in England and Wales and 8.4 in Scotland (Francome 1984, p. 129). There were particular difficulties in obtaining abortions in the Midlands which led to the formation of the Birmingham (later British) Pregnancy Advisory Service (BPAS). This organization was formed in 1968 and by 2002 had a national network of twelve clinics and day care units supported by 35 consultation centres. The organization carries out over 40,000 abortions a year and over two thirds of these are carried out on an agency basis. They are paid for by the NHS but provided free to women. BPAS was represented on the working party which developed the RCOG evidence-based guidelines – *The care of women requesting induced abortion* – and complies with the guidelines recommended quality standards.

The other major charity carrying out abortions in the UK is MSI which operates in over forty countries In 2005 it had served nearly five million clients.

UK law does not give women the right to choose an abortion and this is of concern to a number of people who point out that a women may seek referral from a general practitioner who is anti-abortion and so has problems of access (Bury and Francome 2007). In 2007, a committee of the BMA called for a change in the law so there would be no medical criteria during the first trimester. In 2008 the RCOG stated that the provision within UK law to require that two doctors sign the form for an abortion was anachronistic. It suggested that the signature of only one doctor should be needed (RCOG 2008). These changes would bring British law more into line with that of many other countries which now give women abortion on request. I decided to see whether the people of Britain would support a more liberal law. In September 2013 I commissioned a poll from GFK/NOP. It asked: *Do you think that women should or should not have the right to choose an abortion in the first three months of pregnancy.* In response over three quarters agreed (77 per cent) and just over one in ten (11 per cent) disagreed with the rest (11 per cent) not answering or not sure.

The abortion figures for 2012 show that the rate fell to 16.5 per 1,000 women which is the lowest it has been since 1997 and is a six per cent drop on 2011. They also show that 97 per cent of the abortions were funded by the NHS. Just over a third of these (35 per cent) were carried out in NHS hospitals Over three in five (62 per cent) were carried out by independent organizations – mainly BPAS or MSI – but were provided free to the women. The other three per cent were paid for privately. Just over nine in ten (91 per cent) of abortions are carried out under 13 weeks gestation (Education for Choice 2013). Medical abortions have become more common and currently are nearly half (48 per cent) of all terminations.

Another interesting finding from the 2012 figures is that the number of abortions performed on non-residents was only 5,850 which was a five per cent decline on 2011 and the lowest since 1969. As over four out of five (84 per cent) of the women are from Ireland there has been speculation that increasing numbers of Irish women have been obtaining illegal abortion with pills obtained over the internet (Education for Choice 2013).

Northern Ireland (NI)

The 1967 Abortion Act does not apply to the region. We have seen that many women have travelled to Britian for their terminations. A study by MSI found that 91 per cent of women attending its clinics would have preferred to have their abortion at home (Francome 2004, p. 42). There have been 'two important developments. On 11 October *BBC News* reported 'Marie Stopes private abortion clinic to open in Belfast'. The clinic duly opened one week later and MSI said that it was going to carry out medical terminations up until 9 weeks gestation but were going to adhere to the legal framework. It was to be headed by Dawn Purvis, a former politician (BBC 2012).

The second story raised the issue of whether Irish women should be able to get free abortions like the rest of the UK. I commissioned a poll on this issue. Fieldwork between 13–15 August 2010 found that the majority (52 per cent) of the British population were in favour and two in five (40 per cent) were opposed (GFK). In 2012 the issue was raised in the *Belfast Telegraph* which said that Northern Irish women may get free abortions like the rest of the UK even if they were having an operation that would be illegal in NI. The legal profession refused to support this in 2014 but future developments of the situation remain to be seen.

Conclusion

We have seen that divisions between Eastern Europe and the rest of the countries are quite marked. However, there are signs that change is occurring and in the UK we may expect the number of abortions to decline as modern contraception becomes more widely available. However, there are wide variations in abortion rates even within Western Europe. Some countries have shown great signs of progress. The abortion rate in Italy for example declined by a third in the years 1980–1999, abortions are down by a quarter in Denmark, by a fifth in Finland and also reduced in France and Sweden.

In some respects Europe points the way forward. With good quality contraception, education and access to services the abortion rate can be brought down well below the levels pertaining in societies which are more restrictive in the area of fertility Furthermore, the presence of good services such as AID or *in vitro* fertilization can help women who would otherwise be involuntarily childless.

Europe points the way forward with generally good quality contraception leading to low abortion rates.

Chapter 3
Asia

> 'Every day pregnant women go to the church not only to pray, but to buy abortion drugs from the dozens of stalls that surround it'. (Conde 2005)

Unsafe abortion is a major cause of maternal morbidity and mortality in Asia. Overall, the WHO and the Guttmacher Institute estimate that in the year 2008 the continent had 27 million abortions, a slight increase from 26 million in 2003. The rate of unsafe abortions was unchanged at 11 per every 1000 women aged 15–44. The rate of safe abortions remained around 17–18 per 1,000 women aged 15–44 (Sedge et al. 2012a). (Unsafe abortions accounted for 17,000 deaths in 2008, which was 12 per cent of pregnancy related deaths (WHO 2011, Table 6). Asia's population growth has reduced in recent years. In the period 1970–75 fertility was 5.0 children per woman. It fell to 3.0 in the period 1990–95, 2.3 in 2000–2005 and 2.2 in 2010–2015 (UN Population Division 2014). At this rate it was nearing the rate of replacement. The UN region of Asia includes many countries in the Middle East and those such as Turkey which many would consider to be part of Europe. However, in line with other researchers I shall follow the UN geographical regions. This further divides Asia into four sub-regions which are Eastern, South-Central, South Eastern and Western.

Table 3.1 shows that Singapore had the lowest maternal mortality rate in Eastern and South-Eastern Asia in 2010 at three deaths per 100,000 live births. The second best country was Japan with a rate of five per 100,000. Third lowest was South Korea. The highest maternal mortality rate was that of Laos which has one of the world's highest rates and a rate which is almost double that of the second highest country which is Cambodia. The median rate for Eastern Asia was the rate of 37 for China. The median rate for South Eastern Asia was that of the rate of 59 for Vietnam. The rates could clearly come down a great amount for the countries with the most dangerous childbirth. As far as infant mortality is concerned the lowest rate was for Japan at 2.2 per 1,000. It was closely followed by Singapore. Sri Lanka was third lowest. Once again, the highest rate was Laos, which had over 25 times the Japanese infant death rate. Again, the median rate for Eastern Asia was that of China with a rate of 15.2/1,000). The median rate for South Eastern Asia is that of 18.2 for the Philippines.

Table 3.2 shows that Qatar and Israel had the lowest maternal death rates in Western and South Central Asia. Both countries reported seven per 100,000 live births. The worst rate was that of Afghanistan (460/100,000), followed by Pakistan (260/100,000) and Bangladesh (240/100,000). The median figure for Western Asia is the 25/100,000 of Lebanon and that of South Central Asia is the rate of 67/100,000 for Turkmenistan.

Table 3.1 Eastern and Southern Asia

	Maternal mortality per 100,000 births	Infant mortality per 1,000 births	Population millions
	2010	2013	2013
Eastern Asia			
China	37	15.2	1,349.6
North Korea	81	25.3	24.7
South Korea	16	4.0	49.0
Japan	5	2.2	127.3
Mongolia	63	34.8	3.2
South Eastern Asia			
Brunei	24	10.8	0.4
Cambodia	250	52.7	15.2
Indonesia	220	26.1	251.2
Laos	470	56.1	6.7
Malaysia	29	14.1	29.6
Myanmar	200	46.3	55.2
Philippines	99	18.2	105.7
Singapore	3	2.6	5.5
Thailand	48	15.4	67.4
Vietnam	59	19.6	92.5

Source: CIA 2013, selected pages from p. 1 to p. 780.

As far as infant mortality rate is concerned, the lowest figure was the 4.0/1,000) for Israel with Qatar second lowest (6.6) and Kuwait third lowest (7.7). The highest rate is Afghanistan (119.4/1,000) followed by Pakistan (59.4) and Bangladesh 47.3 The median rate of Western Asia is that of 14.5 for Oman. For South-Central Asia it is 39.5.

The number of unsafe abortions varies a great amount according to WHO figures. Abortion is legal in all Eastern Asia countries and the number of unsafe abortions is negligible. However, in South Central Asia there are yearly 10.5 million abortions, and 17 unsafe abortions per 1,000 women aged 15–44. In South-Eastern Asia there are 22 unsafe abortions per 1,000 women aged 15–44 and in Western Asia, 16 unsafe abortions per 1,000 women of childbearing age (Sedge et al. 2012). In Western Asia almost one in six (16 per cent) of maternal deaths are due to unsafe abortion. However, as measured by the number of unsafe abortion deaths per 100,000 live births, the highest rate is 30, in South-Central Asia. (WHO 2011, Table 6). Unsafe abortion is most dangerous in South-Central Asia, with 200 deaths per 100,000 abortions (WHO 2011, Table 7).

The regional offices of the International Planned Parenthood Federation (IPPF) in South-Asia and in South-Eastern Asia and Oceania have stated their

Table 3.2 South Central and Western Asia

	Maternal mortality per 100,000 births	Infant mortality per 1,000 births	Population millions
	2010	2013	2013
Western Asia			
Armenia	30	17.6	3.0
Azerbaijan	43	27.7	9.6
Bahrain	20	9.9	1.3
Cyprus	10	8.8	0.2
Georgia	67	14.2	4.6
Iraq	63	38.9	31.9
Israel	7	4.0	7.6
Jordan	63	15.3	6.3
Kuwait	14	7.7	2.7
Lebanon	25	14.8	4.1
Oman	32	14.5	3.2
Qatar	7	6.6	2.0
Saudi Arabia	24	15.1	26.9
Syria	70	14.6	22.5
Turkey	20	22.2	80.7
United Arab Emirates	12	11.3	5.5
Yemen	200	51.9	25.4
South-Central Asia			
Afghanistan	460	119.4	31.1
Bangladesh	240	47.3	163.7
Bhutan	180	30.0	0.7
India	200	44.6	1,220.8
Iran	21	40.0	79.9
Kazakhstan	51	22.3	17.7
Kyrgyzstan	71	29.7	5.5
Nepal	170	41.8	30.4
Pakistan	260	59.4	193.2
Sri Lanka	35	9.2	21.7
Tajikistan	65	36.2	7.9
Turkmenistan	67	39.5	5.1
Uzbekistan	28	20.5	28.7

Source: CIA 2013, selected pages from p. 33.

goal is to make abortion rare, safe, legal, and available, and to move forward the liberalization of abortion services. This is a challenge, especially in regard to expanding. The IPPF Regional offices identify the following problems in improving services.

- Reduced efforts to address unsafe abortion due to legal, political, cultural and religious barriers in the region.
- Reducing donor restrictions on funding related to abortion.
- Poor data and documentation of abortion-related issues resulting in limited availability of evidence-based documents for advocating with governments.

Many countries in Asia encounter a lack of capacity in implementing clinical abortion-related services and in effectively advocating the right to access safe abortion. Young people as well as unmarried women are particularly under-served. Where abortion laws are the least permissive, such as in the Philippines, Myanmar, Laos and the Pacific Islands, IPPF suggests it is critical to open up the issue of unsafe abortion to public debate and address the social and cultural mores that stigmatize women who have had abortions.

Unsafe abortion continues to be one of the most easily preventable causes of maternal mortality. Across Asia abortion remains a controversial issue because of social, cultural and religious factors, which often translate into discrimination against women. The situation is exacerbated in South Asia, where entrenched gender discrimination and inequity deny women their bodily integrity and the right to control their fertility. Poor access to reproductive health services and a lack of awareness about the implications of unsafe abortion leads women to experience an inability to make informed decisions on abortion and related services.

A report for the UN by leading Arab researchers became the subject of impassioned debate in 2002. They found that development was being undermined by failings on three major issues. These were first, civil and political freedom, secondly knowledge production and dissemination, and thirdly, the empowerment of women. The failure of women to gain equality has been linked to continued high fertility. The average total fertility rate for the Arab world was 3.4 children per woman, which was high compared to the world average of 2.7 at that time. However, the figure was a great reduction from the average of over six children found in the previous generation (Fargues 2005, p. 43, DeJong et al. 2005). One of the major reasons for the fertility reduction has been the rising age of marriage. Three quarters of women in the 1950 birth cohort married under the age of twenty compared to just a third in the 1970 cohort. The mean age of marriage has risen from under 20 to over 25 in just one generation. Increasing length of education is a crucial factor. The proportion of married women in the labour force in Arab countries was one third in 2000 and it is still not wholly acceptable for married Arab women to work outside the home. However, patriarchal practices are diminishing and changes are clearly going to continue. For larger nations, let us consider the situation country by country.

Afghanistan

> Arguably no other force in modern history has practiced such severe cruelty in its segregation of women from all aspects of the public realm. (Brookes 2005)

In 2000 only 13 per cent of Afghan women were literate. For men the figure was 43 per cent (CIA 2013, p. 2). The country suffers from dark forces who do not wish to see the country benefit from educational development. The country gained its independence from notional British control in 1919. There was an experiment in democracy which ended in a 1973 coup and a 1978 counter-coup. The Russians invaded in 1979 and a destructive war led to the Taliban, a Pakistan sponsored group taking over the capital Kabul in 1996. After the 9/11 attacks the US, Allied forces and the Northern Alliance overthrew the Taliban for sheltering Osama bin Laden. The country has been ravaged by war and its health statistics reflect that. In 2008 it had the highest maternal mortality rate in the world (CIA 2012, p. 1). Over the period 2000–2005 its life expectancy at birth was only 43 years. It increased to 50.1 years in 2013 which is still over 30 years less than the developed countries. Its religion is 80 per cent Sunni Muslim and 19 per cent Shia with only one per cent being of other religions. The average woman was reported by the UN as having 7.5 children 2000–2005 the third highest in the world. However, the number of births was down to 5.6 in 2011 and 5.5 in 2011. This is a reduction of two births per woman and dropped Afghanistan's birthrate to eighth in the world (CIA 2012, p. 1, CIA 2013, p. 1).

Invasions prevented improvements in health for the local population. The infant mortality rate 2000–2005 was 149, and although it improved to 122 in 2011 and 119 in 2013, it was still the highest in the world. It means that every 100 women experience nearly 60 infant deaths during their lifetime.

A problem for the country's family health services came with the election of George Bush. He reinstated the 'gag rule' in January 2001. As stated earlier this meant that no US funds could go to non-governmental organizations that perform, provide information about, or refer for abortions. However, an important liberalization of the position occurred in August 2005 when seven family planning centres opened. In 2009 there were reports that the some Taliban groups were fiercely opposing contraception and that they may use the topic as a pretext for further attacks on health centres (IRIN 2009). However, the Taliban are divided on the subject and some critics also see them as being ignorant of the health and theological implications. For example, Hamdulla Rahmani, a lecturer at Kabul University commented 'The Taliban are illiterate and do not know about the real spirit of Islam … they're wrong' (IRIN 2009). There have been several reports about how Mullahs have been concerned about the high maternal mortality rates and have been calling upon contraception to be used to space births and save lives and also so reduce family size. Katie Drummond commented:

> Another important development was a proposal from the Afghan health minister Suraya Dalil to improve the lot of women. She was quoted in Ms Magazine 'Many Afghan women know about family planning, birth spacing and contraception. They need to have access to them'. (White 2011)

In a separate development MSI set up a meeting with Afghan Mullahs during which the high maternal mortality rate in Afghanistan was discussed and contraceptives proposed. Clearly, many of the deaths in childbirth are relatively easily preventable (White 2011). In 2010, 22 per cent of married women were using a form of contraception.

There are those willing to support change both in education and in the area of reproductive health:

> Legal access to abortion is a necessary element of an overall guarantee of women's rights and autonomy which in turn will aid the eventual development of a viable Afghan state. (Brookes 2005)

When the hostilities end Afghanistan will have the opportunity to bring its social conditions up to the level in the rest of the world.

Bangladesh

In 1901 the Area of East Bengal had a population of 29 million. The name changed to East Pakistan and in 1951 the population of the area had risen to 44 million. East Pakistan broke its relationship with West Pakistan in 1972 and became Bangladesh. The official law did not allow abortion for pregnancy following rape. However, because of rapes by soldiers in 1972 the law was suspended for a period. The population continued to rise to 87 million by 1981 and so the population had tripled in only 80 years. By 2013 the population estimate was 164 million. Nine out of ten residents are Muslim and the other 10 per cent Hindu. The fertility rate has been declining. The average woman had 3.1 children in 2005 but this declined to 2.6 children per woman in 2011 and 2.5 in 2013 (CIA 2013, p. 61).

Contraceptive use increased from 36 per cent per cent in married and cohabiting women in 1990 to 62 per cent per cent in the year 2011, including 52 per cent using modern methods of contraception.

The Bangladesh Bureau of Statistics 2000 data has also shown that one-fifth (21 per cent) of maternal deaths were due to complications from abortion. In 1978 abortion deaths accounted for 26 per cent of pregnancy related deaths. This led in 1979 to a government circular including menstrual regulation in the national family planning programme. (Menstrual regulation is the evacuation of the uterus without a prior pregnancy test.) A national programme was developed to train doctors and paramedics to provide it in all public health facilities. Subsequently, menstrual regulation was included as part of the reproductive health package of services within the national Health and Population Sector Programme and the 1998–2003 five-year national health programme of the Government. Following the completion of this five-year plan the next national Health, Nutrition and Population Sector Plan 2004–2007 addressed the menstrual regulation issues with the same priorities as before.

Menstrual regulation is provided by mid-level health workers as well as by doctors. It is allowed up to 10 weeks from the last menstrual period if performed by a physician and eight weeks if carried out by a family welfare visitor or medical practitioner. They are therefore widely available. In 2010, an estimated 653,000 legal menstrual regulations were performed. The rate of complications is higher than in developed countries because of low-resource facilities and imperfect training. In 2010, some 12 per cent of women having menstrual regulations suffered complications that were treated in health facilities. Despite the existence of legal menstrual regulation services, the Guttmacher Institute estimates that an equal number of clandestine unsafe abortions take place each year. Among the many reasons are that services are not available locally everywhere, some women are unaware of their existence, women are past the gestational limits, or if they are rejected for medical reasons or because providers refuse to serve young women, or those with no children. The complication rate of clandestine abortions may be three times that of legal ones. (Guttmacher Institute, 2012). In recent years, misoprostol has become widely available and will no doubt further reduce the number of unsafe abortion complications and deaths.

Cambodia

The country gained independence from France in 1953. There was a tumultuous period of civil strife during which an estimated 1.5 million people died (CIA 2012, p, 123). However, the elections of 2008 were relatively calm. The capital is Phnom Penh with a population of 1.5 million. The religious background is 96 per cent Buddhist. The birth rate (2011) is 25.2 per 1,000 and the death rate 8.0, which gives a population growth rate of 1.7 per cent per annum. The data for 2011 shows that the average woman had 2.8 children and life expectancy at birth was 63.0 years.

Family planning first became available in Cambodia in 1991 with the contraceptive pill and the condom being the principle methods. Three years later the UNFPA helped the Royal Government of Cambodia to set up a sponsored family scheme, which was followed in 1996 with a mass media campaign. In 1995 the prevalence of modern contraception was only seven per cent, but it increased to 35 per cent using modern methods by 2010/11 and 51 per cent if non-modern methods, such as withdrawal, were included. Even so, there is room for improvement in the family planning facilities.

A liberal abortion law was passed in 1997 that allows abortion on request in the first 12 weeks of pregnancy. However, at that time the cost of a safe abortion was prohibitive. Consequently, a number of women tried to self-induce abortion by such methods as jumping, ingestion of traditional herbs or pills. In more recent years, safe abortion has become available in both public and private facilities. Medical abortion has become widely available. There has been progress in the maternal mortality rate, which has halved in recent years. However, the estimated rate of 250 in 2010 is still way above what it could be (CIA 2010, p. 125). The Asia Safe Abortion Partnership (ASAP) states that many women do not realize that abortion is legal and consequently they seek out 'backyard' providers. A 2006 study suggested that 11.6 per cent of women had abortions at home and a further 32.9 per cent had them in someone else's home. So, almost a half were conducted away from a health facility in potentially unsafe conditions (ASAP 2014).

China

In the year 2013, the population was estimated at 1,349,585,838 the total fertility rate was 1.6 children per woman, and the average life expectancy was 75.0 years, an increase from 59 in 1970. The capital Beijing has a population of 12.2 million. However, the largest city is Shanghai with a population of 16.6 million. China has no official religion but traditional religions include Taoism, Confucianism, and Buddhism. Christians comprise 3–4 per cent of the population and Muslims 1–2 per cent (CIA 2012, p. 150). The population suffered under the autocratic rule of Mao Zedong until 1978 when his successor introduced market orientated development and the GNP quadrupled by the year 2000. In 2010 China became the world's largest exporter (CIA 2013, p. 152).

In 2006, 85 per cent of Chinese women were using birth control and the country was fourth highest in the world in this respect. Its methods tended to be different to Western usage. For example, 29 per cent of women and five per cent of men were sterilized. In addition 41 per cent of women used the IUD. In contrast, only one per cent used the contraceptive pill and nine per cent the condom. The stress was on married women and longer acting methods (Siville 2005).

Abortion was legalized by a directive from the Minister of Health in 1957. Peiping University president Ma Ying-Chu was quoted in the *New York Times* (28 July 1957) as saying that China must attempt to limit its population or face defeat in efforts to industrialize the nation and raise living standards. In a special article Chen Muhua, a vice-president of the People's Republic, stated that China's population had risen from 540 million in 1949 to 975 million in 1978. However, he reported the success in reducing the crude birth rate from 40 per 1,000 population in the 1960s to 18.4 in 1978. He stated that the aim was to achieve zero population growth by the year 2000. He noted that amongst the 17.4 million births, 5.2 million were third or higher order, and if these could be eliminated then the rate of natural increase would be reduced to only seven per 1,000. Muhua also drew attention to the incentives to persuade people to have just one child. These included a stipend until the child was 14 years old and priority in schools and jobs. He commented that the Marxist states had been over critical of Malthus and argued that a rapidly expanding population was detrimental to capital accumulation and affected the standard of living.

In 1979, China introduced the policy that women were to have only one child, with exceptions for ethnic minorities and couples both of whom are only children.

This was to be enforced by financial and educational penalties but not by coercion, and forced abortion and sterilization were against the law. During the period 1973–1978 the number of abortions was relatively stable and only increased marginally from 5.1 million to 5.2 million. However, numbers then rose over the next five years to a peak of 14.4 million in 1983 before decreasing and stabilizing at around 10 million abortions a year. (Henshaw and Morrow 1990, p. 34; Sedgh et al. 2011) The relatively high abortion rate (in the range of 29 in 2008) despite the high level of contraceptive use reflects the very low birth rate and possibly increasing sexual activity of unmarried women, who may not have easy access to contraception.

Although the official view is that women should not be coerced into abortions, the Western media has reported numerous cases where women were forced to have terminations against their will. This may be due to over-zealous local authorities going beyond the national directives. An example was reported by Associated Press (2005): in Linyi, a city of over 10 million people situated around 400 miles SE of Beijing, local authorities reportedly raided the homes of families with two children and sterilized one of the parents. The article also said that women who were pregnant with a third child were forced to have an abortion. Activists on the issue were making attempts at legal redress. The one child policy was more observed in the urban areas than in rural districts.

One problem identified by the Chinese news agency Xinhua, is that many people faced with having one child have preferred it to be male, so that by 2006 it was estimated that 117 boys were born for every 100 girls. Two years earlier there was a report that of 31 provinces, regions, and municipalities in China, all but seven had at least 110 baby boys born to 100 baby girls. This led to a 'care for girls' campaign supported by the authorities. Zhao Baigo commented that the aim was to have a normal sex ratio by 2010 (Xinhua 2004). Comparisons between China and the rest of the world are illuminating and show that this aim has not been met. In 2013 in the age group 0–14 years in China there were 124.8 million males compared to 107.3 million females. So males made up 53.8 per cent of the age group. This compared to 51.4 per cent in the rest of the world. (CIA 1913, p. 806). So compared with the rest of the world 2.4 per cent of girls are missing which is 2.6 million girls aged 0–11 years. The sex imbalance is believed to result from abortion of female foetuses after clandestine amniocentesis or ultrasound examination.

In 2012 there was a great deal of concern when BBC News reported that Feny Jiamei was forced to have an abortion at seven months gestation because she could not afford the fine for a second child. The authorities commented 'such practice has seriously violated the relevant policies set by national and provincial family planning commissions which harmed the image of our family planning work.'

The data for 2007 indicates around 16 million live births and 7.6 million abortions. If this figure is confirmed it will mean about one third (32 per cent) of pregnancies end in abortion (excluding miscarriages as usual). However, reporting is incomplete and the actual abortion rate is probably considerably higher. It might have been expected that the abortion rate would be lower given the high contraceptive usage. However, one factor is that younger women seem to be more likely to have an unwanted pregnancy before marriage, and the reported rate of contraceptive use omits unmarried women.

India

The country gained Independence from the UK in 1947. Violence led to the creation of two states, India and Pakistan. The country is undergoing rapid economic growth. The average woman had 2.6 children in 2013. Its capital, New Delhi, had a population of 21.7 million in 2011. According to the 2001 census the population is 81 per cent Hindu, 13 per Muslim, two per cent Christian and two per cent Sikh (2002 census). The average length of life from birth is 67.1 years (CIA 2012, p. 337).

In 1951 the Government sponsored a birth control programme and since that time has continued to push various measures. One was sterilization, which was particularly encouraged for almost two years until March 1977. During this period 10 million people received a vasectomy or tubal ligation. Many of these operations were compulsory for parents of three or more children. This programme led to the defeat of the government of Mrs Gandhi and was drastically cut back. The National Family Health Survey in 1989–90 investigated contraceptive methods and found that 34 per cent of women chose a permanent method, 12 per cent other methods, while 52 per cent of women continued not to employ any method. This changed, and by the year 2005/06 55 per cent of married women were using contraception. There is also evidence that condoms are being promoted in the country in response to the HIV/AIDs prevention programme and 80 per cent of India's 12 billion, five-year programme was dedicated to promoting condoms. However, there is some opposition and Hindu nationalists have been working for the elimination of sex education in many schools and suggested teaching teenagers yoga instead (p. 2007).

The Indian abortion law had its origins in the British 1861 Act, which arguably made abortion illegal except to save the life of the women. However, the high number of unsafe abortions leading to maternal mortality led in 1964 to a re-evaluation of the situation with the government-appointed Shah Committee:

> Doctors frequently came across gravely ill or dying women who had taken recourse to unsafe abortions. They realized that the majority of women seeking abortion were married and under no socio-cultural pressure to conceal their pregnancies and that decriminalizing abortion would encourage women to seek abortion services in legal and safe settings. (Hirve 2004, p. 114)

The Shah committee carried out a comprehensive review of the law on both medical and compassionate grounds and in 1966 called for a legalizing of abortion. It led to the Medical Termination of Pregnancy Act (1971) that legalized abortion throughout India except for the states of Jammu and Kashmir. The law allowed doctors to carry out an abortion on a variety of grounds including rape and incest, grave risk to the physical or mental health of the woman in her actual or foreseeable environment, when the pregnancy results from contraceptive failure, or on humanitarian grounds. It also allowed abortion for foetal abnormality. The operation can take place in any hospital maintained by the government but requires approval or certification of any facility in the private sector. For abortions up to 12 weeks only one doctor's signature is needed but for 12–20 weeks two are needed, except in an emergency (Hirve 2004, p. 115). Although abortion is legally available in a variety of situations the doctor still has the final approval.

In 1982 S.M. Dasgupta told a population control conference that nearly four million illegal abortions were carried out each year. He called for further liberalization of the law and for women to have abortion on request (*Guardian* 17 February 1982). The Indian Parliament tried to take more control of the situation with new measures including the Medical Termination of Pregnancy (Amendment) Act 2002. It improved some of the bureaucracy surrounding registration and, for example, facilities were no longer required to have on-site capability of managing emergency complications (Hirve 2004, p. 116).

In 2000, the National Population Policy of India was initiated in order to promote family planning. It also recognized the importance of providing safe abortion facilities. Although the act does not deny care to the single or the widowed, divorced and separated, it uses the phrase 'where any pregnancy occurs as a result of failure of any device or method used by any "married" woman or her husband for the purpose of limiting the number of children' (Hirve 2004, p. 117). Some activists have argued for replacing 'married women' with 'all women'. This has not been taken up as it has been argued 'it would imply tacit recognition and sanction of sexual relations among those who are unmarried or were previously married' (Hirve 2004, p. 117). In practice, safe abortion services are generally available to unmarried women, though they often avoid legal services for fear that confidentiality will be breached.

India is similar to China in that there is evidence of abortion used for sex selection. One of the adverts read 'Invest 500 rupees (for a sex test) now and save 50,000 rupees (for a dowry) later'. Renuka Chowdhury, the Minister of State for Women and Child Development stated that the number of girls per 1,000 boys was 945 in 1991 but fell to 927 in 2001 (Page 2007). In 2002, the government banned abortion being used for sex selection. Furthermore, in 2006 the government launched a national campaign with the slogan 'My strength, my daughter'. It also passed the Pre-Natal Diagnostic Techniques Act which aimed to prevent medical staff from telling parents the sex of a foetus. However, the London *Times* carried a full page report in February 2007 on the problems of female infanticide and abortion, stating:

> Police in central India have found 390 body parts from foetuses and newborn babies – thought to be unwanted girls – buried in the backyard of a Christian missionary hospital. Separately the Government said that it was setting up a network of girls' homes – dubbed the 'cradle scheme' – in an effort to stop poor Indians from killing their daughters … Boys in India are traditionally regarded as future breadwinners whereas girls are considered a financial burden.

Mrs Chowdhury commented 'It is a matter of international and national shame for us that India, with a growth of nine per cent, still kills its daughters'. She continued to say that they were telling the people that if they did not want girls they could place them for adoption in Government-financed homes (Page 2007). The estimates for 2013 show that in the age group 0–14 years there are in India 187.2 million males and 165.2 million females. A number of proposals have been made to end sex selection. One was to allow abortion only up until 12 weeks – before the sex could be determined. However, this was countered with the argument that it would lead to illegal abortions in the case of pregnancies over twelve weeks. In fact there is some evidence that the problem is getting worse. In the case where the first child is a daughter the number of daughters born in the next pregnancy was 906 per 1000 boys in 1990. However, in 2005 it had declined to 836 (Boseley 2011).

The Indian economy is growing and this will produce extra resources to improve services. It is also the case that mifepristone and misoprostol are widely available and so the government may have more success in improving services in the future. The abortion reporting system recorded 629,472 abortions in 2010, which is down from a peak of 770,714 in 2001, but because most facilities do not submit reporting forms there are actually several times this many safe abortions. In addition, there are many unsafe abortions with their attendant complications. Among the reasons are women feel more comfortable going to local informal providers such as midwives whom they know than they do going to doctors, even the small fees charged by doctors are a barrier, safe services are not available everywhere, and some women do not know where to go.

The UN estimates that there were about 26 million births per year in 2005–2010.

Indonesia

Indonesia has progressed significantly. Its life expectancy at birth increased from 47 in 1970 to 71.9 in 2013. This suggests a great improvement in social conditions (CIA 2013, p. 342). Indonesia consists of over 18,000 islands, the five biggest being Jakarta, Sumatra, Kalimantan, Sulawesi and Irian Java. The 2000 census found the religion to be 86 per cent Muslim, nine per cent Christian, two per cent Hindu and one per cent Buddhist. The average woman had 2.2 children in 2011 (CIA 2012, p. 343).

The Government has been concerned with overpopulation for some time. In the mid-1980s it began providing free birth control services at public health centres. From 1988, it began to impose charges on more affluent clients to support the cost of the programme. However, services were still largely free for the poor. In 1989 the UN gave its population award to the president of Indonesia. Strictly speaking, abortion is illegal except to save the woman's life or for certain medical conditions. However, there is evidence that some clinics are adopting a more liberal approach. One in Jakarta reported 500 abortions a month while another in Bali reported 7–10 abortions a day (Pangkahila and Pangkahila 2006).

Although the population is nominally Muslim, it does not seem that the sexual practices of the young follow the conservative behaviour of the past. There is a great amount of pre-marital sexual contact, and teenage pregnancy is not uncommon, although exact figures are available (Pangkahila and Pangkahila 2006). The government, however, is looking towards zero population growth in the near future.

There is division amongst Muslim leaders about how long into the pregnancy an abortion should be allowed. The followers of Imam Hanafi allow abortion up to 120 days after conception. However, others say it should be restricted to 40 days (Guttmacher 2008).

In a major report the Guttmacher Institute commented:

> Each year in Indonesia millions of women become pregnant unintentionally and may choose to end their pregnancies despite the fact abortion is generally illegal. (2008)

It continued to estimate that around two million abortions are carried out each year, giving a rate of 37 per 1,000 women aged 14–29. It discussed the millennium goal of reducing maternal mortality by three-quarters between 1990 and 2015 and proposed a four point plan:

1. Improve contraceptive facilities in order to reduce the number of unwanted pregnancies.
2. Educate the young people into the knowledge and use of safe sex.
3. Provide legal abortion safely to the extent allowed by the law.
4. Improve after-care for abortion and work towards it being included in medical education. Doctors should be taught how to perform manual vacuum aspiration.

The report does not mention misoprostol; however, its availability will help to make abortion safer.

Iran

The religious background is 89 per cent Shia Muslim and nine per cent Sunni. Its life expectancy from birth is 70.4 years and the average woman has 1.9 children (2011). The capital, Tehran, has a population of 7.2 million (2009) (CIA 2013, p. 347). Iranian women were amongst the first to work for equal rights in the early part of the nineteenth century. The leaders were, however, repressed. Until 1931, women could not seek divorce; this changed under the pressure from women's organizations, and in 1936 females gained entrance to Tehran

University. Women obtained the vote and the right to stand for election. The educational emancipation was such that by 1978 one third of university students were female. Abortion was restricted by Article 622 of the Islamic Punishment Law which only allowed it to save the life of the woman. After the revolution of 1979 and the increased importance of Islamic law, two stages of pregnancy were recognized. Until 120 days the foetus was considered not to have a soul. Once it was considered ensouled the pregnancy was treated quite differently. In March 2005, *Agence France Presse* reported that the increase in unsafe abortion pushed Iran's conservative leaders to consider a change in the law (Cabatu and Bonk 2005). Consequently, on 5 April 2005, Parliament approved liberalization to include abortion in certain cases including the possibility of birth defects. During the debate one Member of Parliament drew attention to the fact that abortion was not condemned by the Quran. Although the law was passed by Parliament in Iran there are twelve clerical men appointed to a *Council of Guardians* who can overturn a law if they judge it does not comply with Islamic principles. This is what occurred and they maintained 'It is against sharia to abort children who would inflict a financial burden on the parents after birth due to mental or physical handicap.' However, a new law was passed on 31 May 2005 which was approved by the Guardians Council on 15 June (Larijani and Zahedi 2006). Legal medical organizations specified 51 different medical problems for the woman and foetus which could lead to abortion and others could be considered.

After the 1979 revolution, the Islamic government encouraged large families in the belief that a large population would strengthen the country, and the total fertility rate was over 6 children per woman. Then following the war with Iraq, the new Supreme Leader saw that the country would have difficulty providing food, education, housing and employment for the burgeoning population and established a family planning programme that became one of the most effective in the world. The Health Ministry provided a full range of contraceptive methods, including pills, condoms, IUDs, implants, tubal ligations, vasectomies, and post-coital contraception (Wikipedia http://en.wikipedia.org/wiki/Family_planning_in_Iran). Fertility fell to 2.6 children per woman in 1995–2000 and to 1.9 in 2005–2010. Then policy was reversed again in 2006 when President Ahmadinejad called for an increase in population from 70 million to 120 million. In 2010 the government again instituted payment to families for each child.

The family planning clinics are supportive of women who have had illegal abortions. Furthermore, 'Health care providers do not feel compelled to report illegal abortions to authorities' (Larijani and Zahedi 2006). The increased use of prostaglandins for abortions instead of curettage has helped reduce the maternal mortality rate.

One of the practices in Iran that seems alien to many people but affects unwanted pregnancy, is the practice of temporary marriage or sigheh. This practice only applies to Shias, and not Sunnis and seems to have developed when people would be away from home for long periods and it was judged they could not be expected to forgo their sexual needs. President Rafsanjani said in 1990: 'Don't be promiscuous like the Westerners' but use the God-given solution of temporary marriage'. This led to some complaints of inequality as men could not only have four wives, but also unlimited temporary marriages. Ten years later the *New York Times* told the story of Maryam and Karim who had a secret relationship which they carried out in Karim's mother's house for five years (2000). These temporary marriages could be as short or as long as people wish them to be. Maryam and Karim renewed their temporary arrangement every six months so that they could have sex legally and in keeping with their religion. Maryam had been previously married and divorced and this meant she could undergo a temporary marriage without the permission of a male relative. In this case after five years Karim decided to end the relationship and married a virgin. Maryam said that she now planned to look for a permanent marriage. This practice of temporary marriage allows the institutionalization of less committed sexual relationships. Children of such relationships may not have the support of a committed father, but with fertility control using contraception and abortion women may have the necessary control over their fertility.

As of 2005/2010, Iran was one of only a few Muslim countries with a birth rate below replacement level.

Iraq

The country has undergone three major conflicts. It fought a territorial dispute with Iran from 1980–88. It seized Kuwait in 1990 but was expelled. Subsequently, US-led forces invaded the country in 2003 and military action continued until 2011 (CIA 2012).

During the period 2000–2005 the average fertility rate was 3.2 children per woman and this increased to 3.6 in 2011. Life expectancy at birth was 72.4 years in 2011. The population is 60–65 per cent Shia and 32–37 per cent Sunni with Christians comprising around three per cent of the population (CIA 2012, p. 351). Its capital Baghdad had a population of 5.8 million in 2009. An instructive statistic shows the extent of the suffering of the people in Iraq in the domain of health. In 1970 both Iran and Iraq had an average life span of 55 years. However, by the period 2000–2005 the average Iranian lived to 70 years which is nine years longer than the average of 61 years for Iraqis (Wright 2006, p. 488). Fortunately the Iraqi length of life increased to 71 in 2011 (CIA 2112, p. 351). The war has had a disastrous effect on health services and in the first 18 months after the 2003 invasion more than a third of the facilities providing family planning were destroyed. It was estimated that the risk of death was 2.5 times the level before the invasion (Round Up 2005a) One observer reported looting and damage to clinics leading to a decline in family planning and contraceptive services (Majaj 2005). However, despite this there has been some positive change. In 1989 only 14 per cent of Iraqi women of fertile age used contraception, it increased to 44 per cent in 2000, to 50 per cent in 2006 (Index Mundi 2013), and 53 per cent in 2011.

Legal abortion in Iraq is difficult to obtain. It allows abortion only to save the life of the woman and for severe foetal malformation. Furthermore, the operation has to be approved by three medical practitioners plus the woman's husband if she is married. It is therefore not surprising that feminists spoke in 2007 about 'the rising rate of illegal abortion in Iraq. Women who wanted a legal abortion were invited to go to India. An advertisement stated 'The abortion clinic of India operates out of Bangalore, India and offers a safe alternative for women.' It provided a phone number for women to call to make an appointment.

There is evidence that women's groups are becoming more active in pressing for equal rights. The Iraqi Women's Rights Coalition called for numerous changes including:

1. Equal rights of family inheritance.
2. An end to 'honour' killings.
3. The criminalization of rape.
4. The abolition of marriages for girls under 16 and polygamous marriages.
5. The right to abortion up to 12 weeks.
6. The right to equal education and employment opportunities.
7. The right to live alone and travel freely.
8. Right to refuse to wear Islamic veiling (McNevin 2012).

If these measures are introduced they would introduce great change in the social life of Iraq.

Israel

In 2011 the average woman had 2.7 children and life expectancy from birth was 81.0 years. The religious background is 76 per cent Jewish, 17 per cent Muslim (mainly Sunni), two per cent Christian and four per cent other religions (CIA 2012, p. 36). Jerusalem is the capital, but the largest city is Tel Aviv with a population of 3.2 million (CIA 2012, p. 361).

One of the surprising things about the situation in Israel is that the passing of its abortion law was so contentious. It might be thought that given the role of Jews in liberalizing the laws throughout the world the country would have moved swiftly to abortion on request. This is particularly so because we know that in 1952 the District Court of Haifa ruled that abortion openly performed on *bona fide* medical grounds was legal. From that time onwards doctors were not prosecuted and in practice abortion was freely available from medical practitioners. The law in Israel is based on the 1977 Penal Code, clauses 312–321. In the lead up to the Act the issue of abortion divided Israeli society. Feminist groups pressured for women to have the right to choose. They were supported by those on the left, but opposed by the orthodox religious groups, the right wing and the Israeli Society of Gynaecologists. The *Jewish Chronicle* (19 March 1976) reported that a meeting of 500 rabbis proclaimed a worldwide day of prayer to prevent the liberalizing law from coming into being as it could 'spell suicide for the nation'. This kind of argument has a long history and a variant was later used by the British Chief Rabbi (*Jewish Chronicle* 29 January 1982) when he argued that without abortion there would be four million Jewish Israelis rather than three million (Francome 1984, p. 147). He drew comparisons to the murder of Jews by the Nazis. The weakness of this argument is that many Israeli women who had abortions would nevertheless go on to have the number of children they wanted when they felt the time and possibly that their relationship was right. Right wing nationalists argued for the need to increase the Jewish birthrate. Geula Cohen of Herut said 'the only Bill needed is one to encourage the birth rate, not to decrease it' (*Jewish Chronicle* 28 January 1977). She was opposed by the civil rights leader Shulamit Aloni: 'A woman's body is her own. It is not there to serve the army, the State or the nation'. The opposition of the gynaecologists seems to be largely due to the fact that they objected to women feeling they had the right to make them carry out an abortion (Francome 1984, p. 147).

The law that passed in February 1977 was a compromise. The most controversial aspect was the social clause: 'The family or social circumstances of the woman are such that for her to have another baby would be seriously injurious to her or her children'. Political change gave the religious parties more power and led in 1980 to this reason for abortion to be removed. Two years later a leading Jerusalem gynaecologist was quoted as saying the change had had little effect because 'any woman who really wants to terminate her pregnancy will find a way to get it done' (*Jewish Chronicle* 19 March 1982). The law specified that a woman should go before a committee of three people including doctors, a social worker and at least one woman. Requests to the committees for an abortion are normally approved. So the Central Bureau of Statistics reveals that in 2011 there were 20,945 applications to the committees. Approval was granted in 98 per cent of the cases and led to 19,212 abortions.

Government data shows the actual number of recorded abortions in 2003 was just under 21,000. It then declined slightly to 19,500 in 2010. In fact the abortion rate per thousand women 15–45 shows some interesting trends. In 1979 it was 23.2 but then rose to a peak of 25.7 in 1984 despite the removal of the social clause from the law. However, then the rate began to fall. In 1986 it was 18.4, 1995 it was 14.3, and in 2011 only 10.4. This is only two fifths of the peak twenty-seven years earlier (Johnston 2013).

These official figures do not, however, tell the whole story for, as the above discussion shows, women with money are able to afford to by-pass the committee system and pay a private doctor. The UN estimates that the total number of abortions are around 40,000 a year.

Japan

The life expectancy at 84.2 years is one of the highest in the world. Its fertility rate per woman was only 1.4 in 2013. The birth rate was 8.2 and the death rate slightly higher at 9.3. Most Japanese observe both Shinto and Buddhist rites. The capital Tokyo has a population of 36.5 million (CIA 2013, p. 373).

Japan has by far the highest usage of condoms in the world. In 2000, almost half (46 per cent) of Japanese couples used this as their method and it comprised three quarters of Japanese contraceptive use in contrast to five per cent usage worldwide (UN 2004, p. 60). One of the reasons for the high condom use is the fact that the Intra-Uterine Device (IUD) was not legalized until 1974, but more importantly the contraceptive pill was not approved for usage until 1999 – nearly 50 years after introduction in the US. In fact, it might not have been approved then had it not been that Viagra was approved for use after only six months in 1998. The unfairness of elderly men in the Japanese legislature looking after their own interests led to outrage amongst women's organizations. However, the pill has not had the popularity it enjoyed elsewhere. For example, in 2009 the percentage of women 15–49 using the contraceptive pill was only three per cent in Japan compared to 44 per cent in France and 18 per cent in the UK (Hayes 2011).

Japan was one of the first countries to liberalize termination of pregnancy. In 1948 it passed the Eugenic Protection Law which allowed abortion until viability for a broad range of conditions including mental illness, hereditary diseases, leprosy, the health of the woman and pregnancy following rape. One requirement was that the woman should be examined by two doctors but this was abolished in 1952. The time limit was reduced in 1976 to 23 weeks gestation and further on 1 January 1991 to 21 weeks. This later change followed a case in 1988 where a doctor attempted to abort a 16-year-old girl, but produced a live baby for which he neglected to care (Francome and Vekemans 2007, p. 53).

In 1949, the first year after the Act, the number of abortions was 246,000. This doubled in the following year and rose to a peak in 1955 of 1,150,000 operations which was an abortion rate of 55.5 for women aged 15–49. By the year 2,000 the number of abortions fell to 341,000 with a rate of 11.7 per 1,000 women. It continued to fall to an estimated rate of 213,000 in 2010 (Johnston 2013a).

One observer, Dr Kunio Kitamura proposed a number of reasons for the declining abortion rate including the fact that young people were having less sex, that some people were opting to have children instead, that sex education had improved and that there was the availability of emergency birth control if problems did arise (2005).

Kazakhstan

The country, previously called the Kazakh Soviet Socialist Republic, is north west of China in Central Asia. It is 47 per cent Muslim and 44 per cent Russian

Orthodox. Its capital is Astana with a population of two thirds of a million (2009). In 2011 its life expectancy at birth was 69.6 years and the average woman had 2.4 children. The President, Ilyinskaya Nursultan won re-election in 2011 with 95.5 per cent of the vote.

As with a number of other countries linked to the former USSR, there was little emphasis on contraception. In 1974, for example, the country effectively prohibited oral contraception.. This approach began to change markedly in February 1994 when a family planning programme was approved and the medical profession was called on to greatly expand services. The percentage of women using contraception increased from 27 per cent to 46 per cent in 1995 (Francome and Vekemans 2007).

Abortion was re-legalized in 1955 in keeping with other countries in the USSR. The number of abortions was 362,000 in 1983, the first year for which there are records. This represented 49 per cent of all pregnancies ending in abortion (not including miscarriages). In the 1990s there was a determined effort to replace abortion with contraception and the number of abortions declined to 134,000 in 2000, 126,000 in 2005, 106,000 in 2010. At this level there were less than a third of the earlier 1983 figure (Johnston 2013f).

Although abortion is legal, an article says that Muslim girls are afraid of shaming their families and resort to potentially fatal unsafe operations:

> Twenty-year-old Aigal met Nurjan a soldier, last summer. She found it hard to resist his advances 'One time I gave into his urging' She sighed. After that, he began to demand sex frequently, promising that eventually they would marry. In September, she found out that she was pregnant. On the advice of an old friend, she went to a woman who provides illegal abortions at home. 'What else could I do?' said Aigal. 'What would have happened to me if the village had found out about my pregnancy?'. (Dosybieva 2005)

The article goes on to say that Muslim girls living in the South of Kazakhstan face a situation where sex before marriage is strictly forbidden and in some cases the sheets of the marital bed are examined for virginal blood. However, when the girls move to the city they have much more freedom and many more temptations. They want an illegal abortion as its help with anonymity. Aigul said 'I was scared to go hospital, because you need to give your address'.

This evidence shows that the legal abortion figures are an underestimate. However, local experts are unable to provide a figure as to the extent of the shortfall.

North Korea (Democratic People's Republic)

After the Second World War Korea was divided into two parts. The North was founded on 1 May 1948 and came under Soviet-sponsored Communist control. It fought a war with the US-sponsored South from 1950–53 and the enmity between the two sides has not been resolved (Famighetti 1999, CIA 2012, p. 393). The religious background is Buddhism and Confucianism but autonomous religious activities are now almost non-existent (CIA 2012, p. 394). The country's capital is Pyongyang which has a population of approximately two million.

The average length of life was only 52 in 1998, however, by 2013 estimates were that it was up to 69.5 years. In the early years of its existence the country encouraged women to have children in the expectation that the population would increase. There was nursery support and financial help. In 1966 the average woman had 6.5 children. The birthrate began to fall, however, and was 2.5 in 1988 and 2.0 in 2013 (CIA 2013, p. 394).

The IPPF commented:

> According to the Reproductive Health Survey of 1998 conducted by the Population Institute, the abortion rate among married women was 17.7 per 1000 women (MIAR: Marital Induced Abortion Rate). From 1998 to 2001, the MIAR declined from 17.7 to 11.1 following efforts to promote FP services. The most common contraceptive methods are IUD followed by oral contraceptives, spermicides and condoms. (2007, personal communication)

In 2002 there were serious allegations that women in prison were suffering forced abortion and also that infanticide was common. Brook commented 'More and more escapees from North Korea are asserting that forced abortions and infanticide are the norm in North Korean prisons'. Willie Fautre, the director of 'Human Rights without Frontiers' said that several hundred babies were killed in North Korean prisons. Runaways from North Korea told of starvation and forced abortions at a UN enquiry. In addition, one woman was forced to drown her baby in a bucket. The UN said the violations were 'systematic, wide and grave' (Brook 2002). The treatment of women in prison was particularly harsh if the foetus was deemed to be of mixed race. This was usually when a Korean women has had a relationship with a Chinese man (Sheridan 2006).

There is also evidence of illegal abortions especially in the more remote areas. An article about illegal abortion in Hyesan said that a lack of access to contraception and an increasingly sexually liberated culture has led to more women choosing illegal and unsafe abortions in North Korea (Cathcart 2012) The article continued to state that the number of unwanted pregnancies were in part due to the problem of getting contraceptives from China because of a clampdown by the authorities.

South Korea (Republic)

Life expectancy in 2013 was 79.6 years and the fertility rate per woman was 1.2 children which is one of the lowest in the world and is a marked reduction from the figure of 4.7 in 1970 (CIA 2013, p. 398). In 2013, the birth rate per 1,000 was 8.3 and its death rate 6.5. Its capital is Seoul with a population of 9.8

million (2008). A survey in 2010 showed the religious background to be 32 per cent Christian, 24 per cent Buddhist, but over two in five (43 per cent) had no religion (CIA 2012, p. 307).

In 1962, the Government instigated a family planning programme. Contraceptive use increased from 79 per cent in married and cohabiting women in 1990 to 84 per cent in the year 2000 and of these two thirds (67 per cent) were modern methods of contraception (UN 2004, p. 57). In the period 2005–2010 contraceptive use was recorded at 80.0 per cent which is a slight reduction but still well above the world average of 63 per cent (WHO 2012).

Jiyeon stated that in 2005 the estimate of the number of abortions in South Korea were 350,000 which was 80 per cent as high as the number of live births. She stated:

> In a clinic in a fashionable area of Seoul, young women wait for doctors to give illegal abortions. They do so despite the fact that abortion is illegal and has been for many years because the authorities choose to 'turn the other way'. Many public officials want a change in the law but have to face 'pro-life' activists. Kim So-Yoon headed the Government sponsored research into the situation and said that big changes were necessary. The internet seems to have made a difference. One woman wrote 'I am a high school student and would like to get an abortion'. (Jiyeon 2008)

In 2012 Sung estimated the number of abortions to be 340,000. This is slightly below the 2005 estimate but is still high by Western standards. He noted the opposition to legalization and commented 'Deep seated disregard for women's rights is behind recent abortion controversy in Korean society'.

In 2013 a controversial book on abortion in South Korea contained the stories of 25 women and why they decided to have abortions. Many of them experienced grief in making the decision to terminate their pregnancy. A married woman said 'It was the saddest moment of my life'. In giving reasons for their decision many women reported that finance was a problem. A mother of two reported she was having great problem coping with two children as she had to work, which meant she could not provide the care she would have liked. A single woman reported that she could not face the social pressures and did not want to inflict a child being 'a kid with no Dad'. The local representative of the 'Pro-Life' group – Choe Jeong – showed some sympathy for such comments and called for an infrastructure to be put into place to support having a baby (Olsen 2013).

Malaysia

In 2013 the life expectancy at birth was 74 years which is an increase from 62 years in 1970. The average number of children per woman was 2.6. Its capital city is Kuala Lumpur with a population of 1.5 million (2009). It is 60 per cent Muslim.

One in five (19 per cent) are Buddhist and one in ten (9 per cent) Christian (CIA 2013, p. 454).

Before 1966 there was very light usage of contraception – at less than one woman in ten. In that year, however, family planning became the official policy of the country and one of its aims was to reduce the increase in population growth from three per cent per annum to two per cent. The percentage of women (or partners) using modern methods of contraception increased to 26 per cent in 1974, 30 per cent in both 1984 and 1994 and then a further increase to 34 per cent in 2004. In 2004 a further 18 per cent used contraception but not a modern method. For example, nearly one in ten (9 per cent) used the rhythm method and three per cent used abstinence. The increase in usage led in 2007 to the Government saying that the fertility rate was 'satisfactory'.

The Abortion Act 1967 was restrictive and the operation became illegal except to save a woman's life. The Malaysian Fertility and Family Survey carried out research into women's attitudes to abortion in 1974 which showed that 71 per cent agreed with it for rape and 52 per cent for the woman's health. (Takeshita et al. 1986) In 1984 the government announced a new population policy aimed at promoting population growth as part of an emphasis on family life. However, this does not seem to have been successful. In 1989 there were concerns about illegal abortion and one estimate was that the abortion ratio was one to every three live births. The law was changed and the Penal Code Amendment Act provided for legal abortions to be done safely under certain conditions. One of these is that the 'continuance of the pregnancy would involve risk to the life of the pregnant woman or injury to the mental or physical health of the pregnant woman, greater than if the pregnancy were terminated'. This wording is clearly lifted from the British Abortion Act 1967 and as early abortion is always statistically safer than childbirth, there is a strong case for saying that abortion is always legal. However, this point does not seem to have been made in the debate in Malaysia.

Muslims make up a sizeable group of the population and, although the Koran says nothing about abortion, on 9 January 2003 the Muslim National Fatwa Council declared that cloning human foetuses was acceptable as long as the foetus was destroyed within 120 days. Ismail Abraham was quoted as saying that 120 days 'would be in keeping with the view in some sections of Islam that until a foetus reached 4 months it has no soul and therefore can be aborted' (Life Site News 2006). This line of thought could allow a Muslim woman to have an abortion in the early months of pregnancy without transgressing the rules of her faith. In contrast, the Catholic clergy in Malaysia takes a very restrictive view, even of birth control. In 2003 Bishop Anthony Lee of the Diocese of Miri was quoted as saying he 'made it a number one priority to reiterate the Church's teaching against contraception and the whole culture of death' (Meaney 2003).

To discover the ease of access to abortion in Malaysia a journalist contacted six clinics at random. Three of these stated openly that they could perform abortions but the other three were more reticent. A nurse said that one doctor carried out two abortions every day and commented 'Some patients walk in wearing school uniform, accompanied by their boyfriend' (Palmdoc 2006). R Jegasothy of the Malaysian Medical Association made the point that over the previous 10 years they had not had a single complaint it could take up about an illegal abortion occurring. It had a few anonymous missives on the subject which could not lead to action. He suggested that doctors were filling a demand and if they stopped then unskilled operators were likely to take over. He commented 'We do not now hear of women dying after inserting lalong or pineapple stalks' (Palmdoc 2006). Overall, abortion seems to be accepted as part of its overall family planning policy.

Women's organizations are not satisfied with the current law. A spokeswoman for the Woman's Aid Organization expressed concern that the decision was in the hands of doctors. She asserted that women have the right to determine the course of their lives and to decide what happens to their bodies (Thwaites 2011). The International Consortium for Medical Abortion (ICMA) reports that another active women's group is the Sisters of Islam which promotes Muslim women's rights through theological arguments. This group has been a strong promoter of the 120-day ensoulment theory (2013).

Myanmar (Until 1989 known as Burma)

This former British colony gained its independence from the Commonwealth in 1948. The people have had to suffer the fact that its political leaders have been placed under house arrest. However, recently there has been a movement towards more openness (CIA 2012, p. 114). In 2011 the average woman had 2.2 children and life expectancy was 65.2 years. Nine out of ten (89 per cent) are Buddhist, four per cent Muslim and four per cent Christian (CIA 2012, p. 115). The capital city is Rangoon which has a population of 4.3 million (2009).

In 1980 only five per cent of women used contraception and the Government was not supportive. In fact it was not until 1991 that wholesale encouragement was given to contraception for the spacing of births. However, use of modern methods of contraception increased from 32 per cent in 2001 to 38 per cent in 2007 and 46 per cent in 2010. In 2007 usage was higher in the urban areas at 49 per cent compared to only 34 per cent in the rural areas. At this time there was an unmet need for contraception for one woman in five (IRIN 2010).

MSI Myanmar has been working in the country with a limited range of services since 1997. It provides help with HIV/AIDS and gives contraceptive assistance. Until 2006 this concentrated on 'birth spacing' but more recently people have been talking in terms of 'Reproductive Health'. Condoms are freely available in the country and are inexpensive at 0.15 US dollars (2013 prices). Some agencies provide them to clients for free, presumably mainly to prevent the spread of HIV/AIDS. There was prejudice against the condom but our local informant tells us that the 'stigma has been reduced significantly in the past decade'.

Abortion is illegal and local women go to China if they want a termination. In addition there is the Mao Tao clinic set up at the border town of Mae Sot where numerous women travel great distances for family planning and health care. We saw in Table 3.2 that Myanmar has a high rate of maternal mortality. At 200 per 100,000 deaths (2010) it is four times the rate of Thailand and seven times the rate of Malaysia. An important article states that in 2010 abortion was the third leading cause of maternal death and that around one in ten of the deaths were abortion related. The Government National Health Plan aimed to carry out research into the issue. One of the statisticians, Ko Ko Saw commented 'It is good if we can provide information which can prevent the problem of unwanted pregnancy, because it is important in reducing the maternal mortality rate (IRIN 2010).

Misoprostol is now available and if it became more widely known it could help reduce the death rates from illegal operations. A local respondent said that the media is controlled in the area of sexuality and for example 'illegitimate' (pre-marital or out of wedlock) pregnancies are not allowed to be portrayed in films or print media.

Nepal

Situated between China and India, this country had a life expectation from birth of 66.9 years in 2013 which is a substantial increase from an average of 42 years in 1970. (CIA 2013, p. 515). In the period 2000–2005 the total fertility rate was 3.5 children per woman. In 2013 the average family size had declined by over a child per woman to 2.4 (CIA 2013, p. 515). Four out of five (81 per cent) people are Hindu and one in ten Buddhist (11 per cent). The capital city is Kathmandu with a population of nearly one million (2009).

Contraceptive use increased from one in five (21 per cent) married and cohabiting women in 1990 to one third (33 per cent) in the year 2000 and of these three in ten (29 per cent) were modern methods of contraception (UN 2004, p. 57) By the period 2005–2010 almost half (48 per cent) of women 15–49 or their partners were using contraception (WHO 2012).

Women in Nepal have historically had a difficult time. In 2001 it was one of three countries in the world where the life expectancy of women was below that of men. An article published in 2001 reported a Nepalese woman saying: 'To be born a daughter is ill fate' and it reported that four out of five women could not read. Furthermore, four out of five homes had no running water (Opesto 2001). The 2001 Nepal Demographic and Health Survey found that one in five births were unwanted and a further 14 per cent were unplanned. Illegal abortion was common and very dangerous. Overall, one estimate was that around 4,000 Nepalese women died of abortion related causes each year and that this constituted half of all maternal deaths (Uprety 1998) More recently some things have improved. For example, in the 2010 census 73 per cent of men and 48 per cent of women were literate (CIA 2013, p. 515).

The headline of an article released by BBC News was *Abortion Nightmare in Nepal* (Singh 2004). This described how in 2000 Shanti Shresta had a problem with her pregnancy. She already had three children and was in her fourth month when she developed a migraine and took paracetamol. She commented further 'I knew instinctively I was miscarrying … my underclothes were drenched in blood'. She was taken to hospital by her landlady who had the responsibility of reporting such a miscarriage to the police. The police saw her as potentially aborting herself and at the hospital she had four armed policeman as guards. This was a waste of resources. 'I was so sick there was no reason for them to guard me. I could not run anywhere.' Her two teenage daughters were left with her husband who was a taxi driver. She was taken to prison and her five-year-old son accompanied her. Although she was not unintelligent, she was illiterate. Consequently, she could not read the paper the police presented to her and signed a confession and was sent to prison for twenty years. Her son was placed in care. Not surprisingly she was deeply traumatized by the event. Fortunately, when the law was changed in 2002 she was released. She commented 'I thought I was going to rot in jail. I never thought I would be released'. However, she had still not been reconciled with her son at the time of the report (Singh 2004).

This experience was by no means unique. In the 1990s nearly 100 women were in prison for having abortions. Not one man was convicted for abortion related activities in the whole history of the Act (Uprety 1998). As a high percentage of pregnancies end in spontaneous abortion which cannot be proved there were probably many women wrongly imprisoned under the law which was later rescinded. On 14 March 2002 the national parliament of Nepal passed a law to legalize abortion for women under 12 weeks gestation. For the period up to 18 weeks gestation abortion was to be legal in the case of rape and incest. In the case of risk to the health of the woman or a disabled foetus there was to be no time limit (Singh 2004). The law was not retrospective and, although some women were released early in April 2003, a report stated that over 50 women were still languishing in prison. However, in 2004 the King declared an amnesty for abortion offences (Singh 2004).

At the beginning of 2011 a court case – Lakshmi Dhikta *v* Nepal was reported. The woman concerned was pregnant for the sixth time and could not pay the required fee of around $20 for abortion and continued to term. The Supreme Court ruled that the Government must provide women with access to safe and affordable abortion services (Centre for Reproductive Rights 2011).

In 2011 there was an estimate that there were 95,000 abortions. This is not particularly high for a country with a population of nearly 30 million nevertheless there was a moral panic about it. B. Rijal, a gynaecologist, said 'The increase in abortions is causing a public health distaste in the country'. Chanda Karki was quoted 'More and more teenagers resort to abortion. In our clinic we get girls under the age of thirteen' (Asia News 2013)

However, others have seen abortions in a different light. MSI reports that there has been a marked decline in maternal mortality rates which fell from 539 in 1996 to 380 in 2008. Table 3.2 shows that in 2010 they were down to 170. K. Thopa commented 'when abortion became legalized in Nepal poor women no longer had to resort to life threatening techniques like drinking poisonous remedies or pushing substances such as bleach into the uterus' (MSI 2013).

On 26 September 2013, the Centre for Research on Environmental Health and Population Activities based in Katmandu celebrated eleven years of the abortion liberalization. It said that the Nepal Government had initiated several important steps to guarantee legal abortion. However, it commented that there was still much work to be done as a survey showed only 56 per cent of women (2011) knew a place where they could obtain a safe abortion service.

Pakistan

In 2013 life expectancy was 66.7 and it had increased from only 48 years in 1970. In 2013 the average woman had 3.0 children. In 2000–2005 the total fertility rate had been 4.0 children per woman so there has been a substantial fall. The religious background is three quarters (75 per cent) Sunni Muslim and one in five (20 per cent) Shia Muslim. Its capital is Islamabad with a population approaching one million. The largest city is Karachi with 13 million people (2009). (CIA 2012, p. 552).

The Family Planning Association was set up in 1953 and following the International Conference on Population and Development in Cairo in 1994 the Government instigated programs for birth control. The Population Welfare Division planned that over the five years 1993–8 the population increase should reduce from 2.9 per cent to 2.6 per cent per annum. By the year 2003, the rate of increase had been reduced to 2.1 per cent and I 2011 it was down to 1.6 per cent (Wright 2006, p. 483). Contraceptive use increased from one in eight (12 per cent) married and cohabiting women in 1990 to one in three (33 per cent) in the year 2000; 23 per cent used modern methods of contraception (UN 2004, p. 57) There was then a levelling off and in 2006–7 contraceptive use was only 30 per cent (Vlassoff 2009). Data from the WHO (2010) indicate that contraceptive use from 2005–2010 was 27 per cent. This is well below the world average, despite the fact there are no religious difficulties in use the use of contraception. The Koran for example, encourages women to breastfeed extensively which can help with the spacing of births. However, there are problems in spreading the message because the wives who would like to use contraception are often in an inferior position within the family compared to their husbands and mother-in-law. They may want her to have more children.

MSI began working in the country in 1992 and Dr Laila Shah, its Medical Development Team Leader, at the time said in 2007:

> Contraceptive usage is relatively low in Pakistan. This is due to 'poor access to family planning services, to the cost of these services, the fear of side effects, myths and misconceptions about family planning methods'.

However, Dr Shah did note some cause for optimism in that knowledge of family planning is high and condoms are readily available (Personal communication 2007).

Until 1990 the abortion law was based on that developed by British colonialists in India in 1860. This was very restrictive especially after the period of 'quickening' – about four months into the pregnancy. In 1989 the Pakistan Supreme Court found the law to be invalid as not in keeping with the principles of Islam. This led in 1990 to a new law which allowed abortion for 'necessary treatment'. This is not clearly defined. It retained the idea that there should be differences between abortion being carried out after four months in line with Islamist teaching that after this time the limbs and organs are formed and the foetus has a soul.

An investigation of the situation in Pakistan in 2002 by the Guttmacher Institute assessed that the abortion rate was 29 per 1,000 women and that overall there were 900,000 abortions a year. It revealed that pregnant women were often forced to visit illegal clinics run by midwives and that 23 per cent of these abortions resulted in the women being hospitalized for complications. The report also suggested that men should become more involved in fertility control (Population Council 2007).

In the geographical areas where international groups are operating there is clearly much better access to a wide range of family planning services. The Guttmacher Institute reported that amongst poor, rural women only seven per cent obtained their abortions from recognized doctors and 42 per cent used *dias* (traditional birth attendants). In contrast, amongst better off women in the urban areas, 49 per cent were attended by doctors and only nine per cent by the dias. Dr Shah also said:

> We are already providing FP services through 47 delivery services. These include all family planning methods including surgical ones, we also offer TSIC which stands for Treatment for Septic and Incomplete Abortions in all our centres.

The International Pregnancy Advice Service (IPAS) is providing training in manual vacuum aspiration to government and private doctors and as this early treatment fits in well with the tenets of the Muslim religion, it could prove acceptable. In addition, medical abortion is freely available using misoprostol.

Philippines

In 2013 the average woman had 3.1 children. This is a reduction from 4.3 in 1985–1990 (Juaraz et al. 2005). Life expectancy at birth has been increasing and while in 1970 it was 57 years, in 2013 it was 72 years (CIA 2013, p. 577). The religious background is over four out of five (83 per cent) Catholic, The capital city is Manila with a population over 11 million. (CIA 2012, p. 574). Kate McGeown writing an article with the title 'Fierce debate over Philippine contraception bill' comments:

> In one of Manila's sprawling slums, Clarita is busy making lunch for her family. She has ten children and making sure they do not go hungry is a daily struggle. Down a narrow alleyway another desperately poor woman has eight children. Another woman just around the corner has nine. Not surprising then that the Philippines has the highest birth rate in South East Asia. In 1990 there were 60 million Filipinos. Now there are more than 95 million. Clarita is Catholic. She regularly attends church and has a picture of Jesus Christ and a bible verse taped on to the wall of the one small room in which the family live, But recently she has begun to think that on one matter at least the Church is wrong. (2011)

She disagreed with Church's opposition to contraception. Contraceptives are available in the Philippines. The contraceptive pill is sold over the counter and there are many outlets for condoms. However, they are very expensive. So the President Benigo Aquiro III introduced a bill providing poor people with free family planning advice and contraception. It was known, in shorthand, as the R.H. Act (Reproductive Health). The Catholic bishop Fr Bacani attacked it with spirit:

> It is not the business of government to be promoting contraceptive services. It is like the Government saying it will pass a law which will fund the promotion of pork eating amongst Muslims.

The Bishop was supported by a well-known person in the Philippines, a former boxer turned politician Manny Pacquiao, who said that 'Contraception is against God's will'. However, his position was compromised somewhat when his wife told the media that she had been taking the pill for many years. The R.H. Act was eventually passed and in 2013 the *Huffington Post* (1 March) commented the 'Philippines contraception law points to the Catholic Church's waning power. The law was the bishop's worst nightmare. They no longer sway the masses'. In March 2013 the Act was delayed by the Supreme Court.

We await developments.

The abortion law in operation is the revised Penal Code of 1930 which officially makes abortion illegal except to save the life of the woman.

The large Catholic majority has restricted the development modern contraception. Dr Diego Danila of the Department of Health said that attempts to address unsafe abortions through initiatives like more vigorous family planning are opposed by the Church. Conde, writing in the *International Herald Tribune*, said that Filipino politicians only speak about abortion to condemn it but that meanwhile 'more and more women are dying'. Furthermore, foetuses are often dumped in the environs of churches. However, it is not clear to observers whether this is because it is in order to secure eternal life for the supposed soul or whether it is to punish the Church for its hard line attitude (Conde 2005).

Official estimates are that there are 400–500 thousand unsafe abortions a year. The WHO puts the number much higher at 800,000 abortions. This would be the highest rate in Asia. Jean Marc Olive, the WHO local representative, estimates that

70 per cent of unwanted pregnancies end in abortion. Over one third (36 per cent) of women are pregnant before marriage and the local 'pro-life' group estimates that one in four pregnancies ends in abortion. Olive commented on a survey of attitudes to births 'families it seems would like at least one child less than they have' (Conde 2005).

An important study of the incidence of abortion was carried out by Juaraz and colleagues (2005). They obtained data from 1,658 hospitals and estimated that 78,900 people were hospitalized in a year for post-abortion care. They estimated 473,400 women had abortions giving a rate of 27 per 1,000 women aged 15–44. One third of the abortions were carried out by doctors or nurses and two thirds by traditional practitioners. One quarter of the hospitals in their study stated that the after effects of abortion were one of the ten major causes of admission (Juaraz et al. 2005).

One of the centres for the distribution of abortifacient pills is the Quiapo Catholic Church in the capital Manila. Conde comments 'every day pregnant women go to the church not only to pray but to buy abortion drugs from the dozens of stalls that surround it'. The church he comments has 'become almost synonymous with abortion' (2005).

Anti-abortion leaders confirm that the problem exists and are concerned about the high level of abortion. The leader of the Philippines 'pro-life' group – a nun called Pilor Versoza – commented about the trade: 'We would assign volunteers to chase after women who had just bought from vendors and tell them about their options'. The group also put up a sign telling women there were alternatives to abortion; however, it was pulled down (Conde 2005). The bestselling abortifacient is Cytotec (misoprostol). The drug was made illegal but is still on sale for a price of just below one dollar a pill. The right to life group says that the pills are smuggled in from South Korea and Bangkok.

Juaraz and colleagues comment that the high number of abortions in the country is part of a generally restrictive social and political climate. This has suppressed the development of modern forms of contraception and resulted in people using withdrawal methods and periodic abstinence. This leads to unwanted pregnancies and abortions. They suggest that there is a shortfall in services and that around half of women of reproductive age need effective contraception (2005).

Saudi Arabia

In 2013 the average life expectation at birth was 75 years and the average woman had 2.2 children which is substantially down from 3.8. in 2000–2005 (Wright 2006, p. 665, CIA 2013, p. 635). So the average woman was having over one and a half fewer children than ten years earlier. Its religious background is almost one hundred per cent Muslim and most of these are Sunni. The capital city is Riyadh with a population of 4.7 million (2008). Muslims from around the world are encouraged to visit the city of Mecca at least once in their lifetime, if they can afford it. Medina also has great religious importance (Wright 2006, p. 665).

The economy is to a large extent based on oil which constitutes 55 per cent of its GDP and produces 80 per cent of Government income. Shops and restaurants close five times a day for prayers. No citizens are allowed to convert from Islam to another religion and other religions are not allowed to have public meetings. The society is strongly divided by gender and women in particular are subject to many restrictions. After their first menstrual cycle they must dress in a long black cloak called an abaaya. They are not allowed to drive cars nor ride bicycles, especially in the cities. Women are rarely allowed to testify and in the Sharia court the testimony of one man counts as equal to that of two women (USA Bureau of Democracy). Women are not allowed to marry non-Muslims, however, men can marry Christians and Jews. An unusual practice for Sunni Muslims is the practice of 'Al-Mesyar (or short day time visit) marriages where the woman forgoes maintenance rights. There are no restrictions on the number of these that a man can contract and they are in addition to his official wives (Ottoway 2004). Women only make up five per cent of the work force but there was a slight liberalization in 1997 when they were given the authorization to work in the hotel industry. Women are not allowed to travel alone nor with a man who is not a relative. They are not allowed to attend hospital unless accompanied by a male relative or with written permission and so clearly women cannot seek birth control or abortion. In the year 2000, 20 Saudi women obtained abortions abroad but this number declined to eight in the year 2005 (Johnston 2007a). There are external pressures for Saudi Arabia to liberalize its restrictions. However, these seem to be resisted and Amnesty International's report into the country reported a lack of co-operation from the authorities (2003).

Despite the problems the birthrate has declined and there is evidence of increasing contraceptive use. A cross sectional study of 225 women at day care centres in the Al-Quassim region found that married Saudi women were keen to space their children and delay another pregnancy for two or three years. Overall 45 per cent of the women had been using contraception for over a year. Seven out of ten had been using the pill, one in eight the IUD and one in fourteen condoms. The better educated women were twice as likely to be using contraception compared to the less educated. Many of those who did not use contraception said that children were a blessing from God (Sheeha 2010).

There is evidence of illegal abortion. In one case two Filipino women were sentenced to two years imprisonment and 700 lashes. They were alleged to have been carrying out abortions for three years and charging $930 (Associated Press 1999).

'Sarah' an American woman went to Saudi to work when already pregnant. She had a female boss who had previously also had an unwanted pregnancy. Her boss advised her to go Mumbai for a safe operation. This she did and commented 'The complete procedure was painless, in fact pleasant for I had received an anaesthetic shot for the first time in my life. The next day I flew back to Riyadh to rejoin work.' This statement was used by an Indian abortion advertisement to encourage more Saudi women to travel to Mumbai.'

So it seems that Saudi women may well be moving to the Irish solution where they provide little or no service at home but rather force their women to travel overseas.

Sri Lanka

The country became independent from Britain in 1948 and had the name Ceylon until it was changed to Sri Lanka in 1972. There was a civil war with the Tamil Tigers and a great deal violence and allegations of war crimes. The Government forces declared that it had defeated the remnants of the Tamil army in 2009. The average length of life from birth is 76 years (2013). The average woman has 2.2 children. Seven out of ten (69 per cent) of people are Buddhists and the others are largely Christians (6 per cent), Muslims (8 per cent) or Hindu (0.7 per cent) The capital city is Colombo, 700,000 in 2013).

Sri Lanka was one of the first developing nations to understand the importance of investing in human resources and promoting gender equality. As a result, it has achieved health and education outcomes more consistent with those of high-income countries. For example, of all the thirteen countries in South-Central Asia it is the only country with an infant mortality rate below one per cent and its rate is below half of that of the second best country – Uzbekistan. It also liberalized its economy in the late 1970s ahead of other developing nations and maintained healthy economic growth despite the devastating 20-year civil conflict. However, on the negative side, 90 per cent of Sri Lanka's poor continue to live in rural areas where access to basic services is limited.

Sri Lanka has undergone significant family change and the average age of marriage has increased. For women the average was 18.1 years in 1901 but increased to 24.6 years in 2000, so it rose by 6.5 years. In 1998 education was made compulsory for the 5–14 years age group (de Silva 2003). An important development in the country occurred on 23 December 1997 when a Population and Reproductive Health Policy was approved by the National Health Council chaired by the Prime Minister. It had eight goals. It aimed to produce a stable population, safe maternity, sex equality, and responsible behaviour, increased responsibility towards the welfare of the elderly, promotion of the economic benefits of migrants, increased public awareness of health and an improved population policy.

MSI has been active in the country since 1973 and is partly responsible for the large increase in contraceptive use. Currently MSI is in partnership with the local organization Population Services Lanka. It aims to provide birth control services even in 'far flung villages' and reported that in 2002, 66 per cent of couples were using contraception and 44 per cent were using modern methods (MSI 2007A).

As far as abortion is concerned the Penal Code of Sri Lanka is based on an 1883 law which permits abortion only to save a woman's life, making abortions performed under any other circumstances a criminal offence (de Silva 2003). Studies suggest that a high prevalence of abortion exists in the country. IPPF estimated that there are 237,000 abortions year (2013). US Aid commented that, although terminations are illegal, 'Abortion services have always been provided at private hospitals and clinics and occasionally at Government hospitals' (de Silva 2003). According to the Ministry of Health, women argue adverse emotional and psychological risks, for example, severe depression and suicidal tendencies, to the well being of the pregnant woman, and many are able to secure abortions at private or government hospitals. In these instances there is little or no government enforcement of the law. On 3 May 2006, anti-abortionists carried out a prayer vigil outside the Marie Stopes Centre in Colombo. They were led by Eshan Dias, President of Cultura Vitae who offered to pray for the doctor's conversion to Catholicism.

There have been attempts from Parliamentarians, women's groups and others for reform of the law. As long ago as 1973 the Medical Legal Society proposed the law be broadened to legalize abortion for such things as the woman's health, rape and foetal abnormality. However, no action was taken. IPPF stated that a number of groups are vigorously continuing their efforts to change the law and that the FPA Sri Lanka has proposed a number of measures to help get safe legal abortions. This includes publicizing the maternal mortality rate, research into non-use of contraception, monitoring attitudes to a change in the law, obtaining statements in favour of liberalization from prominent people and working with the media to promote a liberal agenda (IPPF 2013).

Syria

The country has been suffering the effects of civil war. The hostilities began in March 2011 and estimates put the death toll over 10,000. The country is 75 per cent Sunni Muslim. The president elected in 2007 was Bashar al-Assad a member of the minority Alawi sect. The protests began in March 2011 in the southern province of Da'ra with calls for the legalization of political parties and the abandonment of arrests without charge. The Government has made some concessions such as approving laws permitting political parties. However, calls for Assad to step down have not been agreed. The violence continues as of September 2013.

Figures from the World Bank indicate that in 2009, 54 per cent of women aged 15–49 were using contraception. This was a reduction from 58 per cent in 2006 (2010).

As far as abortion is concerned, it is officially illegal except where there are concerns for the health of the woman or the foetus. However, there have been strong calls for it to be allowed if the woman has been raped. Syrians called upon Saudi clerics to issue a fatwa allowing raped women to have abortions. It led to a heated debate. Buthaina Khalil of the Family Protection Association said that if a woman has been made pregnant because of rape the shame is so great that often she cannot tell anyone. Consequently, she is left to use traditional remedies including boiled water containing aspirin, violent massage and lifting heavy objects. The Muslim religion has less of a doctrinal rigidity than the Catholics and different clerics take different positions. As discussed earlier for those who believe ensoulment comes after 120 days gestation there is little problem.

In an important article entitled 'The black market of abortion in the Arab world' Shadoud quoted a pharmacist in the largest city Aleppo:

> A husband came to me aged 51 years with his wife, 41 years. They had a family of ten and their economic conditions were really bad. He asked for abortion pills saying that his wife was pregnant by accident and that they both did not want another child. I told him that as a pharmacist I could not give abortion pills without a prescription. He begged me citing financial difficulties, so I promised to help, calling up a friend who is a doctor. It cost him $8.00 to get rid of the baby. Although, she would have paid no less than $100 at a doctor's office. (Shadoud 2009)

It is to be hoped that medically assisted abortion will increase and therefore make such incidents less common.

Thailand

It is the only Southeast Asian country to have escaped being taken over by a European power. In the 1960s the average woman had over six children and the Government started to sponsor family planning. Now the average woman has 1.7 children, which is well below replacement level. Life expectancy at birth in 2011 was 73.8 years which is an increase from 58 years in 1970 (Wright 2006, p. 482). The capital is Bangkok with a population of 6.9 million (2009).

Contraceptive use was high at seven out of ten (71 per cent) married and cohabiting women in 1990 and rose only slightly to 72 per cent in 2000, Over the period 2005–2010 contraceptive use increased to 81 per cent which is fifth highest of ninety-nine countries in this study (World Bank 2013).

The abortion law in operation is based on sections 301–305 of the Thai penal Code of 1956. Under it abortion is legal to protect the woman's health or rape or incest. The law is not, however, rigorously enforced and in the 1970s there were an estimated 300,000 illegal abortions (Population Division 2007). The methods of abortion, it seems, have been either a traditional abortion massage or intra-uterine injections.

The first large scale study of abortion occurred in 1999 and reviewed the records of 787 hospitals. It found that, although abortion was not legal for foetal problems, it was nevertheless often carried out. In fact it found that just over half the abortions performed in government hospitals were illegal under the terms of the Act. So, 34 per cent had an abortion for congenital abnormality, 12 per cent for socio-economic reasons, and five per cent for HIV infection. Just under one per cent had an abortion because of the risks of contacting *rubella* (Warakamin 2004).

In 2004 Whittaker estimated the number of unsafe abortions at 200–300 thousand a year. Further in-depth research by Whittaker studied 164 women of reproductive age in rural areas and 19 others who had had an illegal abortion. She found wide support for a liberalization of the law and that it was the poorer workers who were most at risk of complications because they were more likely to use untrained practitioners (Whittaker 2002). A 42-year-old woman told of her experience:

> I first tried to induce abortion with an injection but after five days I had no menstruation so I paid to go to a midwife. She used an iron rod to abort. I was afraid so I returned home and instead asked my husband to massage and stamp on my stomach. I also bought some medicines that are very hot but still I did not abort. (Francome and Vekemans 2007, p. 63)

With women facing such obstacles to safe treatment there is obviously pressure to change the law, but Whittaker proposes that while at one time the focus was on abortion and health, more recently the notion of reproductive rights is increasing being used to argue the case. The first moves toward liberalization occurred in 1973 and in 1981 a bill was passed in the House. However, religious opposition prevented it from passing in the Senate. In recent years a network of groups have been working together to produce change. These include women's groups, journalists, academics and public health officials (Whittaker 2003).

The extent of illegal abortion is difficult to calculate but one estimated at least 150–200,000 a year. There was concern in 2010 when 2,000 aborted foetuses were discovered in plastic bags at a temple and photographs in the media ensured the incident received great publicity (Palatino 2010).

An article in the *Thailand Times* mentioned that other similarly placed countries – Cambodia, Vietnam and Nepal had the right to choose an abortion in the first three months of pregnancy. However, it suggested that the religious beliefs made such a development unlikely (Editorial 2011).

Turkey

The country has been having accession membership talks with the EU since 2005. It is almost 100 per cent Muslim – mainly Sunni. Its capital is Ankara with a population of 3.8 million. The largest city is Istanbul with a population of 10.4 million. Its length of life from birth is 73.0 years(2013) This is a substantial increase from 57 years in 1970 (Wright 2006, p. 489). The family size in Turkey has shown a rapid decline. In 1990–95 there were 3.8 children per woman, but in the years 1995–2000 it had reduced to 2.5. In 2013 the average woman had 2.1 children (CIA 2013, p. 741). In 2012 the right-wing Prime Minister Recep Tayyip Erdoğan called for women to have a minimum of three children each.

The country legalized contraception in the 1960s. However, there was a tendency for a high proportion of women to use traditional methods. In 1982 the Government adopted a population policy to provide family planning as part of a plan to improve family health and welfare. From 1936 the abortion law restricted legal access to protecting the life or health of the woman or on the ground of foetal abnormality. The growing number of illegal abortions was a factor in leading to abortion and sterilization being legalized on 24 May 1983 under the Population Planning Law. Abortion is now allowed on request in the first 10 weeks of pregnancy under a law which also authorizes general practitioners to terminate pregnancies. After 10 weeks abortion is allowed to protect the life or health of the woman and for foetal impairment. After 10 weeks two doctors must be involved in the decision. One must be an obstetrics and gynaecology specialist and the other a doctor in another field. The woman must get her husband's consent for an abortion and single women must have the approval of their guardian (Population Division 2007b).

In 1974 the Turkish Fertility Service found that 34 per cent of Turkish women had had an abortion and in 1983 the Turkish Population and Health Survey found that 37 per cent of those ever married had had at least one abortion. The 2003 the Turkish Demographic and Health Survey pointed out that 24 per cent of ever married women had had an abortion and of these 58 per cent had had only one. A 2001 study proposed that improved contraceptive advice around the time of the abortion could substantially reduce repeat abortions, and so lower the overall rate. The authors reported, for example, that some providers were reluctant to insert an IUD after an abortion on the grounds that it might interfere with the normal blood flow and they might not be able to determine whether the abortion was complete (Senlet et al. 2001). We have seen that one of the reasons why abortion is relatively accepted is that Muslim religious scholars in the region predominantly believe abortion can be legal for the first 120 days of a pregnancy.

The high rates of repeat abortion led the Ministry of Health to initiate a pilot study into post-abortion family planning. This took place in the Zekai Tahir Burak hospital. At the start of the study in 1991, 65 per cent of women were given post abortion contraception. The researchers tried a four-part plan to increase the uptake. These were improved facilities, improved staff attitudes, accurate information about the wide range of abortion services and finally, they improved the range of contraceptives on offer. They expanded the range of services to provide the contraceptive pill, the IUD, tubal ligation, vasectomy, implants and injectables. The take up of contraception rose from 65 per cent in 1991 to 97 per cent in 1992. They then expanded the study in 1994 to include 10 more hospitals, one of which dropped out. They found that six of the nine new hospitals increased their take up of post-abortion contraception to over 90 per cent and that there were significant changes in methods even in the first six months. The use of IUDs more than doubled to 49 per cent and tubal ligation increased to 15 per cent. The abortion rate in Turkey has reduced. However, several of its East European neighbours continue to have very high rates. This led researchers to comment

'The post abortion programme experience of Turkey can provide valuable lessons' (Senlet et al. 2001).

In the early 1990s an attempt was made to introduce medical abortion. Mifepristone was officially approved in 1994 at which point the Commission approved a study to gather data on medical abortion supported by the Population Council for terminating a pregnancy up until 56 days after last menstrual period. It aimed to test the efficiency of 200 mg mifepristone taken orally at the clinic and then two days later 400mcg misoprostol taken orally either at home or at the clinic. During the study period 470 women were eligible and they could choose a medical or surgical abortion. There were 209 medical abortions and 149 surgical ones and the average length of pain was the same for both groups at between three and four days. Nine out of ten women having a medical abortion said that they would prefer it again compared to seven out of ten of those having a surgical abortion. The authors concluded that the findings supported the introduction of early medical abortion (Akin et al. 2005).

In 2012, Prime Minister Erdoğan caused an uproar. A report said he described abortion as 'tantamount to murder'. This angered women's rights groups and sparked an intense debate. The Istanbul Feminist Collective reacted angrily. It staged a sit in outside the Prime Minister's office and held banners declaring 'Murder is male violence, abortion is a choice' and 'our womb, our life our decision'. The women were supported by the Turkish Medical Association (TTB) who said that if abortion were banned it would lead to illegal operations and an increase in the Maternal Mortality rate. H. Yilmaz, a lawyer and director of the Centre for Legal Support for Women said 'making a decision regarding one's own body is a fundamental human right'. The Committee for the elimination of discrimination against women maintained that denying services which only women needed, including abortion services amounted to sex discrimination and the violation of international human rights.

The pressure seems to have paid off and Nurettin Canikli. an AKP Lawmaker. stated 'The abortion issue is off the agenda. No legislation will be introduced to the parliament on this issue' (*Guardian*, 1 February 2013).

Uzbekistan

The country gained its independence in 1991 and is the third most populous country from the fragmented Soviet Union. The country has exhibited a declining family size. During the period 1985–1990 the total fertility rate was at 4.4 children per woman (Population Division 2007c). In 2013 it had declined to 1.8. So, family size has declined by more than half. Over these years life expectancy from birth has increased from 70 to 73.0 (CIA 2013, p. 781). The country is 88 per cent Muslim and most of these are Sunnis. In addition, nine per cent are Eastern Orthodox Christians and there are three per cent adherents to other religions. The capital is Tashkent, with a population of 2.2 million (2009) (CIA 2012, p. 781).

Its law before independence followed the abortion law of the rest of the USSR and it was legalized a second time in 1955. The law currently allows abortion on request up to twelve weeks and up to 28 weeks on more restricted grounds. In the period it was part of the Soviet Union it had a relatively high abortion rate. In 1971 there were 156,000; in 1981, 166,000 and they rose to a peak of 258,000 abortions in 1988 which is a rate of 61 per 1,000 women of childbearing age. By 1991 – the year before independence – it had reduced to 189,000 which is an abortion rate of 39 per thousand women 15–45 years. In the year 2,000 the number of abortions had declined dramatically to 62,000 with a rate of 9.7 per 1,000 women of childbearing age. By 2005 the number was 47,000 with a rate of 6.5 per 1,000 and in 2010 the number was down to 39,000 which is a rate of around 5.4 per 1,000 (Johnston 2013n). This rate is only one tenth of the level of the peak in 1988 and is much below that of the Netherlands.

The maternal mortality rate showed evidence of some reduction and it declined from 39 per 100,000 births in 1988 to 30 in 2008 (Population Division 2007e). Table 3.1 shows the latest available figure in 28 for 2010 (CIA 2013, p. 780).

So the country has had a reduction in both the birth and the abortion rate which suggests there must have been an increase is contraceptive use and effectiveness. The Uzbekistan Demographic Health Survey (1996) found that 89 per cent of women knew of at least one contraceptive method and 40 per cent were using a method which was provided free of charge. Of those using a method fully 87 per cent used the IUD. There were two other relevant findings from the study. One was that women in rural areas had an average of one birth more than women in urban areas. The total fertility rate was 3.7 children per mother in rural areas and 2.7 in urban ones. The second was that 96 per cent of women breastfed and they kept it up for long periods. In all, 98 per cent of those having abortions already had children (Digest).

The high usage of the IUD was discussed in an article in 2007 entitled ‘Constrained contraceptive choice: IUD prevalence in Uzbekistan’. It discussed the fact that 73 per cent of married Uzbek women had ever used an IUD compared to only 14 per cent who had used a condom. It suggested that in the Soviet area there was one contraceptive choice which was abortion and now there is also one and it is the IUD. The article quotes a nurse in Tashkent that women get given the IUD after the birth of a child ‘regardless of what her mother-in-law, her husband or she wants’ (Barrett and Buckley 2007).

Vietnam

The country was colonized by France in the nineteenth century. The French were defeated by communist forces in 1954. The country was divided into the communist north and non-communist south and the US tried to bolster the south. It failed and signed a cease fire agreement in 1973. Two years later the communists overran the south and united the country. It has been much more peaceful but there have been some regional protests. Four out of five (81 per cent) of people have no religion but nearly one in ten (9 per cent) is Buddhist (1999 census). In 2013 the average woman had 1.9 children which is a slight reduction from 2.2 in the period 2000–2005. The Government has a two-child policy and this seems to have been achieved (Wright 2006, p. 489; Thinh 2009). The average length of life from birth in 2011 was 72.6 years (CIA 2113, p. 792). Contraceptive use is high with 80 per cent of women being covered (World Bank 2012).

There was no written law allowing or prohibiting abortion in Vietnam between 1945 and 1962. In 1962, with the revision of the Law on Protection and Care of People's Health, abortion was made legal in the country. It seems the first year official figures for the number of abortions were produced was in 1978, when there were 70,281 reported. In 1987 the official level was reported at 811,000 rising to a peak of 1.4 million in 1993. At which time the abortion rate was 81 per 1,000. The numbers then reduced. In 2000, 688,000 were reported which is around a 50 per cent reduction from the peak (Johnston 2007g, Chinoy 2007). In part this may have been because of a programme of action started in 1994 which called for governmental and religious organizations to expand contraceptive facilities. During the 1990s, high levels of abortion translated into an average of 2.5 abortions during a woman's reproductive life (Ganatra et al. 2004, p. 105). In 2008, the number of abortions were estimated as 332,000 at which level the rate would be a relatively low figure of 16 per 1,000 women (Johnston 2013f). However, Thinh suggests that the number could be underestimated because some abortions will be carried out in non-public health facilities and others might be pre-marital abortions and not recorded (2009). On the other hand, a WHO report stated that there was evidence that many women who thought they were having abortions were not, in fact, pregnant. It advocated that a history should be taken and there should be a pelvic examination to establish pregnancy. If it could not be established then a urine test should be made. The WHO report also recommended that facilities should not be paid on a fee for service basis for this was likely to encourage unnecessary operations. One problem to which the report also drew attention was the fact that at the time of an abortion the opportunity to discuss future contraception was rarely taken up. If this were changed the number of repeat abortions could be reduced (WHO 1999).

> IPPF commented on the current situation that it was time for the government to energetically raise the abortion issue in the country and implement programs to reduce abortion rates and human suffering (Personal communication)

Yemen

North and South Yemen were divided but united in 1990. There was, however, violence which led to the UN calling for peace. Elections in 2012 led to the choice of a new president (CIA 2012, p. 811). During the period 2000–2005, the average woman had 6.0 children. This was a reduction from 7.7 in 1992. The figure for 2013 is 4.3 children which is a reduction of over three children per family compared to the 1992 data (CIA 2013, p. 811). The average length of life from birth is 64.5 which is relatively low but is a substantial improvement. The capital city is Sanaa at 2.2 million people (2009) (CIA 2012, p. 811).

In part the birth rate reduction may have been due to the National Population Strategy begun in 1991. However, overall, its reduction in fertility is slower than in other Arab countries. One reason might be due to the tradition of early marriage: in 1985 the average age of marriage for girls was 13 years. The infant mortality rate in that year was 156, which means that at the time the average woman had more than one child die before the age of one year. The Government passed a law in 2009 to increase the minimum age of marriage to 17 for females and 18 for males. However, the Sharia Committee argued in October 2010 that early marriage was better. For example it said that it helped prevent breast cancer (Action Now 2012). There have been those working for a new future and in 2011 the Nobel Peace prize was awarded to Tawakko Karman for her 'non-violent struggle for the safety of women' (Action Number 2012). However, there was a great amount of opposition to change and an article published at the end of 2012 was entitled 'After the Arab spring Yemen's women are left behind' It drew attention to the fact that 12-year-old Aisha was wedded to a 30-year-old man one month after her first period. She said that sex was very painful. Other facts were that four out of five women were illiterate and that there was only one woman in the 301 member parliament (Giovanni 2012).

When contraception was developing in the country it was first practised in the urban areas to a greater degree. So in 1991–2, 28 per cent of married women in urban areas used modern methods of birth control compared to only six per cent in the rural areas. However, in 2007 it was reported that only 10 per cent of women 15–44 used modern methods of contraception (Population Division 2007f). A number of observers talk about the country having widespread abortions, but we have not seen any local estimates as to numbers. The country has been receiving help from outside agencies. MSI started to work in the country in 1998 and has been providing services since that time. In 2005 Pathfinder International started a five-year programme of reproductive, maternal and child health. In February 2006 the British Government promised three million pounds extra aid to help cover a withdrawal of funds from the US. Another new development in March 2007 was the agreement made between the Ministry of Planning and International Co-operation and the UN Family Planning Association to set up a population reduction programme for the period 2007–2011. This entailed improving contraception as well as other developments (United Press International 2007).

MSI reports that it is the largest family planning organization in the country and that it served over 400,000 people in 2012 through its network of 15 centres, two outreach teams and 180 midwives. (MSI 2013b).

Abortion is mainly used where women have had their desired number of children. The most popular contraceptive method used is the pill. This fact may encourage women to seek out misoprostol if they need an abortion.

Conclusion

The overall population of Asia was 3.9 billion (2011). Family size varies greatly between countries with 2013 figures showing the average number of children to be 1.2 in South Korea and 5.5 in Afghanistan (CIA 2013, p. 1; p. 398).

The country analysis of Asia shows that women in the region make great use of abortion to control their fertility. It is clear that contraceptive services are underdeveloped in many countries. Consequently a more vigorous approach could reduce the number of abortions and improve women's health.

Chapter 4
Africa

> 'I failed to withdraw because I was enjoying myself. She cried that I had impregnated her. She then checked the calendar to note the date and time that I had impregnated her.'

Africa has particular problems in the area of sexual health. One local observer pointed out that in countries south of the Sahara, pregnancy is a great risk to women. The death rates were over 50 times that of the US. An article in the *International Herald Tribune* (15 December 2011) was called *Africa's Abortion Wars*. Okeowo pointed out that South Africa (up to 12 weeks) and Cape Verde (up to 14 weeks) were the only two countries in sub-Saharan Africa to have liberal abortion laws. Brookman Amissah (2003) stated:

> It is not by custom that Africans are against abortion, rather it is the colonial laws that we need to reform. Many former British colonies still have the long discredited 1861 Offences Against the Person Act and former French colonies such as Mali have the Napoleonic code making abortion illegal.

We will see that 45 African countries signed the Maputo Treaty which pledges to relax laws.

As far as contraception is concerned usage is generally low. In 2008 for example less than one in five (17 per cent) married women in sub-Saharan Africa were using modern contraceptive methods. However, we will see that there have been signs of increased use (IRIN 2011).

Estimates for the year 2000 were that there were 4.2 million unsafe abortions in Africa with a rate per woman aged 15–44 of 24 per 1,000. The number of deaths from unsafe abortion was estimated to be 29,800 with the UN calculating a case fatality of seven per 1,000 unsafe abortions (UN 2004, p. 89). This is the highest in the world and about seven times the rate for Latin America and the Caribbean (UN 2004, p. 89). A later estimate is that each year the number of unsafe abortions in Africa has increased to around 6 million with 30,000 deaths (Okeowa 2011).

Africa's population growth has reduced in recent years. In the period 1970–75 it was an average of 6.7 children per woman. It fell to 5.6 in the period 1990–95 and to 5.3 from 1995–2000 (UN 2004, p. 29). Further falls have been identified in the country by country evidence.

One important development in Africa was the first ever regional conference on unsafe abortion in Addis Ababa in 2003. This brought together 112 people which included Ministers of Health, policymakers and media representatives. It called on governments to review restrictive laws and to provide increased funding for programmes which addressed unsafe abortion. The Conference was co-convened by the African Partnership for Sexual and Reproductive Health and the Right of Women and Girls. The organization's objectives include the promotion of bodily integrity, healthy reproduction and the right to live free of coercion violence or punishment related to sexuality or fertility (Hessini 2005, p. 91). Also in 2003 the African Union adopted a protocol on the rights of women in Africa. It called for states to protect women's rights by authorizing abortion in the case of sexual assault, rape, incest, foetal impairment or where the pregnancy would endanger the mental or physical health of the woman (Hessini 2005, p. 92).

A first round in the liberalization of laws occurred in the 1970s – Zambia (1972), South Africa and Namibia (1975), Liberia and Zimbabwe (1977). In the 1980s there were changes in the Seychelles (1981), Ghana (1985) and Cape Verde (1986). In the 1990s liberalization occurred in Botswana (1991), Seychelles again (1994), Burkina Faso, South Africa again (1996) and in 2004 in Ethiopia. Kenya and Egypt liberalized their laws in 2010 Rwanda in 2012 A movement towards more restrictions occurred in Equatorial Guinea in 1991 (UN 2004, p. 88).

Regardless of the law, safe abortion services can be obtained by women with sufficient financial resources. In some countries only a few women are able to access these services while in others safe services are widely available. We will now consider the situation in the larger African countries. In all there is a country analysis of 32 of the countries below:

Eastern Africa Burundi, Comoros, Djibouti, Eritrea, Ethiopia, Kenya, Madagascar, Malawi, Mauritius, Mozambique, Reunion, Rwanda, Somalia, Uganda, United Republic of Tanzania, Zambia, Zimbabwe.

Middle Africa Angola, Cameroon, Central African Republic, Chad, Congo, Democratic Republic of the Congo, Equatorial Guinea, Gabon.

Northern Africa Algeria, Egypt, Libya, Jamahiriya, Morocco, Sudan, Tunisia, Western Sahara.

Southern Africa Botswana, Lesotho, Namibia, South Africa, Swaziland.

Western Africa Benin, Burkina Faso, Cape Verde, Côte d'lvoire, Gambia, Ghana, Guinea, Guinea-Bissau, Liberia, Mali, Mauritania, Niger, Nigeria, Senegal, Sierra Leone, Togo.

The following table lists the maternal death rate by society. In part this reflects the number of unsafe abortions which contribute towards the level. The table also gives details of the infant mortality rates. These will reflect both the quality of social conditions as well as the level of medical care.

Table 4.1 shows both Somalia and Chad had high maternal mortality rates estimated at 1,000 and 1100 per 100,000 births. These rates are well above the death rate for Mauritius which is only 60. For Eastern Africa the median country is Zambia with 440 maternal deaths per 100,000 which is less than half the level of Somalia but is still over seven times the level of Mauritius. The median figure for

Table 4.1 Eastern and Middle African Countries

	Maternal mortality rate per 100,00	Infant mortality rate per 1,000	Population millions
	2010	2013	2013
Eastern Africa			
Burundi	800	58.9	10.9
Eritrea	240	39.4	6.2
Ethiopia	350	58.3	93.9
Kenya	360	42.2	44.0
Madagascar	240	46.1	22.6
Malawi	460	77.0	16.8
Mauritius	60	10.9	1.6
Mozambique	490	74.6	24.1
Rwanda	340	61.0	12.0
Somalia	1,000	101.9	10.3
Uganda	300	62.5	34.8
Tanzania	790	45.1	48.3
Zambia	440	68.6	14.2
Zimbabwe	570	27.3	13.2
Middle Africa			
Angola	450	81.8	18.6
Cameroon	690	58.5	20.5
Central African Republic	890	95.0	5.2
Chad	1,100	91.9	11.2
Congo DR	540	74.9	75.5
Guinea	610	57.1	11.2

Note: Maternal mortality rates based on deaths per 100,000 women aged 15–44. Infant mortality based on deaths in the first year of life per 1,000 live births.

Source: CIA 2013.

middle Africa is that of the Guinea with 610 deaths per 100,000 births. The lowest figure is that of 450 for Angola.

As far as infant mortality rates are concerned, again the lowest rate for the 14 countries of Eastern Africa is Mauritius with only 10.9 deaths per thousand in the first year of life. Again Somalia has the highest rate at 101.9 per 1,000, so over one in ten children died in the first year of life in 2013. The median figures for Eastern Africa was 58.3 for Ethiopia which was lower than that of Middle Africa which was Congo DR (74.9). These death rates are over ten times typical European ones.

Table 4.2 Northern, Southern and Western Africa

	Maternal mortality rate per 100,00	Infant mortality rate per 1,000	Population millions
	2010	2013	2013
Northern Africa			
Algeria	97	22.6	38.1
Egypt	66	23.3	85.3
Libya	58	12.3	6.0
Morocco	100	25.5	32.6
Sudan	730	54.2	34.8
Tunisia	56	24.1	10.8
Southern Africa			
Lesotho	620	51.9	1.9
Namibia	200	45.6	2.2
South Africa	300	42.2	48.6
Western Africa			
Benin	350	58.5	9.9
Burkina Faso	300	78.3	17.8
Côte d'Ivoire	400	61.7	22.4
Gambia	360	67.6	1.9
Ghana	350	39.7	25.2
Guinea	610	57.1	11.2
Liberia	770	70.9	4.0
Mali	540	106.5	16.0
Mauritania	510	57.5	3.4
Niger	590	88.0	16.9
Nigeria	630	73.0	174.5
Senegal	370	53.9	13.3
Sierra Leone	890	75.0	5.6
Togo	300	48.3	7.2

Note: Maternal mortality rates based on deaths per 100,000 women aged 15–44. Infant mortality based on deaths in the first year of life per 1,000 live births.

Source: CIA 2013.

For Middle Africa the lowest infant mortality rate was the 57.1 for Guinea and the highest was the rate of nearly one child in ten (95.0 per 1,000) for the Central

African Republic. These figures show great potential for improvement. Table 4.2 provides details for countries in Northern, Southern and Western Africa.

If we take the countries from the three regions together we see that the maternal mortality rate is highest in Sierra Leone with an estimated 890 deaths per 100,000 births. The second highest rate is Liberia with 770 deaths and the Sudan with 730. The lowest death rate is that of 56 for Tunisia. The median rate is that of 360 maternal deaths in Gambia.

As far as infant mortality is concerned the highest rate is in the former French colony of Mali where estimates for 2013 indicate over one in ten children died in the first year of life. Its rate is over eight times the rate of Libya which is 12.3 per 1,000 live births. The median rate are those of 53.9 deaths per 1,000 of Senegal.

These death rates are so much higher than those of European countries and show clearly that much needs to be done. As far as the maternal mortality rates are concerned a change in the laws to reduce the rates of unsafe abortion would clearly play a large part in improving maternal health and also in allowing women to space their children or choose to have as many as they can look after adequately.

The Maputo Protocol

In March 1995, a meeting organized by 'Women in Law and Development in Africa' called for a protocol to address the rights of women. They took the view that these had been marginalized in the context of human rights in Africa. They commented that women need 'an internationally binding instrument protecting their rights' (Make every Woman Count 2011). It took until 11 July 2003 for the protocol to be adopted by the African Union at Maputo, Mozambique and on 25 November 2005 the required number of 15 states ratified the treaty and the protocol entered into force (Unicef 2006). It was signed (but not necessarily ratified) by the heads of 46 of the 53 countries in the African Union. By January 2013, a total of 36 countries had ratified it.

Ten of the main articles in the Protocol are as follows:

1. Elimination of discrimination against women.
2. Elimination of female genital mutilation.
3. Access to justice and equal protection before the law.
4. Protection of women in armed conflicts.
5. Right to education and training.
6. Health and reproductive rights.
7. Right to a healthy and sustainable environment
8. Rights of inheritance.
9. Special protection of elderly women.
10. Special protection of women with disabilities.

(Make Every Woman Count 2011).

By May 2013, only four countries had neither signed nor ratified the protocol. These were Botswana, Egypt, Eritrea and Tunisia. We will now consider developments country by country in Africa.

Angola

It obtained its independence from Portugal in 1975 and its population was estimated at 18.6 million in 2013. Its capital is Luanda which had a population of 4.5 million in 2009. Its religion was almost half (47 per cent) indigenous beliefs, around two in five (38 per cent) Catholic and one in seven (15 per cent) Protestant. In 2011 its birth-rate was 39.4 and death-rate 12.1. This leads to a growth in population of 2.8 per cent. It average length of life at birth was 54.6 years (CIA 1912, p. 18).

Angola's first 27 years of independence were dominated by the destruction caused by the civil war which ended in 2002. The infrastructure was so badly affected that health care was very poor. For example, at the end of the civil war the maternal mortality rate (MMR) was estimated to be between 1,281 and 1,500 per 100,000. Six years later it had halved to 610. Health is still a big problem, for example in 2011, over a quarter of all children died before their fifth birthday (Makamure 2012).

The law on abortion followed its Portuguese predecessor in being restrictive. Abortion is only officially allowed to save the life of the woman and then only during the first trimester. However, observers have suggested that sometimes an abortion is carried out in hospitals in order to protect the health of the woman.

The general restrictiveness of the law has predictably led to a great number of unsafe abortions. One estimate is that 40 per cent of women who have an illegal operation die of its effects. This seems very high compared to elsewhere but concern for the health of women was one of the factors leading to the Justice Minister G. Prata presenting legislation to liberalize the law in 2011.

Catholic bishops opposed the change. They drew attention to the fact that when Pope Benedict visited Angola in 2009 he warned Africa not to 'promote abortion as a form of maternal health care'. In 2011 the Catholic bishops voted for restrictions. Archbishop Jo Queiroz of Huambo was quoted 'Abortion is not a right for a woman to decide if a human being can or cannot live. Women are responsible for conceiving or not.' (Makamure 2112). There is of course a debate as to whether Catholics should think they should be able to impose church doctrine on a population when it will lead to great harm to women as they have unsafe operations.

Algeria

Its population was estimated at 35.4 million in 2011 and the average woman had 1.7 children which is a remarkable reduction from 2.5 children in 2005 (Wright 2006, p. 481, CIA 2012, p. 9). Despite a civil war, the life expectancy of the country had grown from 53 years in 1970 to 71 years in 2000–2005 and 74.7 in

2011 (Francome and Vekemans 2007, p. 72, CIA 2012, p. 9). The infant mortality rate also showed an improvement and fell from 37 per 1,000 in 2000–2005 to 24.9 in 2011. This is a reduction of around a third in less than a decade. Its religion is 99 per cent Sunni Muslim.

Algeria gained its independence from France on 5 July 1962. Its first free multiparty elections were held in 1990 and were won by the Islamic Salvation Front. This was poised to take control when the army seized power and postponed a return to democracy. This led to civil war and in a 'night of terror' in August 1967 when Muslim fundamentalists killed over 300 people. One estimate is that civil strife and assassinations claimed the lives of 70,000 people between 1992–98 (Chelala 1998). In April 1999 the army reached an accord with the Islamic Salvation Front in return for an end to the uprising.

The violence of the civil war had an important affect on abortion practice. According to the Algerian Criminal Code of 8 June 1966, abortion was only legally allowed to save the life of the woman. This was extended so that as of 2012 it also allowed abortion on the grounds of the woman's physical and mental health. One study of a psychiatric ward found that 30 per cent of women admitted for attempting suicide did so after unwanted pregnancies (Hessini 2007, p. 81). In the period 2005–2010, 61 per cent of women in fertile years between 15–49 used birth control.

Algeria still does not officially allow abortion for rape. However, during the civil war there were many cases of raped women becoming pregnant. On 4 March 1998 the rape attacks led to the Algerian Government successfully asking the religious authorities to declare a fatwa allowing raped women to have abortions. Four days later on International Women's Day, thousands of women protested for change in the law. This has not so far been implemented even though the Government told the UN that it allowed abortion for rape (Hessini 2007, p. 77).

Leila Hessini (2007, 2011) drew attention to the fact that during the period 2000–2005 there were 1,076 deaths from illegal abortions. She commented 'in the Maghreb women need reproductive rights'. The three largest countries of the Maghreb are Algeria, Morocco and Tunisia. She stated that 5.5 per cent of maternal deaths in Algeria are due to illegal abortion. She commented that in many ways Tunisia and Algeria are similar in that they are both former French colonies with Muslim populations and similar economic development. However, Algeria had twice the level of pregnancy related deaths and she commented 'Legal abortion saves women's lives'.

Burkina Faso

The population was estimated at 17.3 million in 2012. In 2011 its life expectancy was 54.1 years; this is a substantial increase over the period 2000–2005 when it was 47 years. Its religion is 60 per cent Muslim, 19 per cent Catholic and four per cent other Christian. It also has 15 per cent Animist (CIA 2012, p. 111). In the year 2011 the birth rate was 43.2 per 1,000 and the death rate 12.5. This gives a rate of natural increase of 3.1 per cent. Its infant mortality rate was estimated at 79.8

in 2011 which is an improvement from 121 per 1,000 births during 2000–2005 (Wright 2006, p. 477, CIA 2012, p. 112). In 2011 the average woman had 6.1 children and so for every 1,000 women there were almost 500 infant deaths. The capital city is Ouagadougou with a population of 1.8 million in 2009 (CIA 2012, p. 112).

Contraceptive use has not been widespread. One problem is that the country followed French law and the banning of contraception in 1920. This was changed in 1986. Still by 1990 only six per cent of women were using contraception. This increased but only to 13 per cent in 2000 (UN 2004, p. 5).

The abortion law was liberalized in 1996. However, it is only legal when it presents risks to the woman's life, or in cases of rape, incest and foetal malformations. While a number of family planning needs remain unfulfilled, constraints in accessing quality services often leads to unwanted pregnancies and illegal abortions, with unpredictable implications for the life of clients. One researcher observed that where 'abortion is restricted, women are obliged to resort to unsafe procedures which can result in many complications and expensive treatment' (Storeng 2011). This theme of the cost of abortion to poor women was taken up by Drabo who followed up 20 women who had had complications following incomplete abortion. Two of the patients died. The others often had delay of treatment while they sought finance to pay the hospital. One woman wanted to keep her pregnancy a secret from her mother. However, she needed money and so had to send a message home for help. She was denied treatment for eight hours until the money arrived (Drabo 2012).

A study by Rossier (2004) and colleagues used a new method of estimating the number of illegal abortions. She observed 'People were not willing to talk of their own abortions but very willing to talk about those of others'. So she set up a research programme in the capital in which she asked a random sample of the population in the fertile age range (15–49) about their friends and relatives with whom they had a close relationship. In the end they sampled 963 women and 417 men of whom 44 per cent named a confidant in the age range. They were informed about 163 illegal abortions which they calculated to represent a total rate of 1.1 abortions for the average woman during her lifetime. These were carried out by the woman herself in 26 per cent of cases, six out of ten (61 per cent) were carried out by a medically trained person such as a nurse and around one in eight (13 per cent) by a traditional healer. One third of the abortions were by injection, one fifth by dilation and curettage and one in eight by household drugs. The other third was not specified. Sometimes people had to make several attempts before the abortion was successful and Rossier and colleagues quote one man who said that first his girlfriend tried tablets but they were too bitter. He gave her money for roots but they also did not work. Consequently he said:

> I took my girlfriend to another healer. I paid 6,000 FCFA (about $9). She told me she was feeling it was coming out, we were all glad and then nothing. I said

> if we did not hit hard, things were going to become difficult. I explained the deal to my friend who repairs mopeds, who talked to other friends. They took him to Latfitenga. He scouted the place for me and two days later he and my girlfriend and I took off (to have an injection in Latfitenga).

The injection achieved its purpose. The increased use of misoprostol has in recent years reduced the need for less safe options both in procuring abortions and also to evacuate the uterus after an incomplete abortion. A study of 100 women given misoprostol after incomplete abortions found that all but two had a complete evacuation of the uterus. Virtually all were satisfied with their treatment (Blandine 2012).

Burundi

The population was estimated at 10.6 million in 2012 and its life expectancy at birth was 59.2 years. Its religion is two-thirds Christian – largely Catholic. Around a quarter follow indigenous beliefs (animism) and 10 per cent are Muslim. In the year 2011 the birth rate was 40.6 per 1,000 population and the death rate was 9.4. This gives a rate of natural increase of 3.1 per cent. The average woman has 6.1 children which is the fifth highest in the world (2012, p. 119).

Burundi is situated in Central Africa and 85 per cent of the population is Hutu, 14 per cent is Tutsi with one per cent being pigmy (CIA 2012, p. 119). Its capital is Bujumbura with a population of 455,000 (2009). Burundi's first democratically elected president was shot in October 1993 and this led to almost twelve years of conflict where 200,000 people were killed. In 2005 a new constitution was agreed and a Hutu dominated Government was elected. The current President was elected in 2010.

The WHO was critical of Burundi in 2001 and argued that its restrictive policy on abortion led to a high number of unsafe operations and many deaths. It argued that as men were the ones who caused the pregnancies then education about contraception should also be directed at them. At this time the war was still running and so there were limits as to what could be achieved.

The end of the dispute meant that more energy could be spent in improving living conditions. The Government announced that it would increase the expenditure on health from eight per cent in 2011 to 15 per cent in 2015 with a focus on the health of women and children (Pathfinder 2012a).

Cameroon

The population was estimated at 20.1 million in 2012. Its life expectancy at birth was 54.7 years in 2012. Its religion is 40 per cent indigenous beliefs (animist)

20 per cent Catholic and 20 per cent Muslim. In the year 2011 the birth rate was 32.5 per 1,000 and the death rate 11.7. This gives a rate of natural increase of 2.1 per cent. It is situated in Central Africa and has many ethnic groups, two official languages (English and French) and 24 major African language groups. In 2011 the average woman had 4.1 children (CIA 2012, p. 127).

Contraceptive education in Cameroon is inadequate according to Schuster and helps explain why unwanted pregnancies occur. Contraceptive use increased from (15 per cent) married and cohabiting women in 1990 to (20 per cent) in the year 2000. Of these less than one in ten (8 per cent) used modern methods of contraception (UN 2004, p. 57). A a consequence, contraceptive use was low and furthermore adolescents' access to education and information on sexual matters including contraception were largely restricted because of the fear of encouraging immoral or unrestrained sexual behaviour' (Schuster 2005, p. 132). As far as married women are concerned, evidence suggests a heavy reliance on the rhythm method. However, gender roles enjoin women to be submissive. Furthermore, one study stated that female respondents 'used dubious methods such as drinking saltwater immediately after sexual intercourse' and even when they had access to modern contraception the risk of pregnancy was high because of their lack of knowledge about correct usage (Schuster 2005, p. 132).

More recent research confirms the lack of knowledge and only three in ten (29 per cent) women who were sexually active used contraception and only just over three in ten (32 per cent) knew how to protect themselves against HIV/AIDS. One problem for the country is that the medical system has a disproportionate Catholic input. There are 28 Catholic hospitals and 235 clinics. At these facilities contraception is not available and after sex birth control is not provided even for rape. The Church authorities advised women to continue with their pregnancy and then place their child in a Catholic orphanage. Some local observers propose that the Catholic Church went beyond the law in attempting to stifle reproductive rights. Contraceptive use is low and between 2005 and 2010 it was only 29 per cent (World Bank 2012).

A positive development for women's rights in Cameroon came in May 2009 when the Government ratified the Maputo protocol. Abortion is legal in Cameroon to save the health or life of the pregnant women and in the case of rape. In addition there are well equipped clinics which carry out abortions openly for women who can afford it. Clandestine abortions are carried out by a variety of people including trained midwives, so called native doctors and lay abortionists. Prosecutions for illegal abortion are rare and it seems that women are more concerned about the public shaming that could occur if the abortion became widely known (Schuster 2005, pp. 130–2).

Cameroon clearly has a need for better education, an improvement in services to the poorer groups who cannot afford good treatment and a change in the law so that all can access safe, treatment within the law.

Chad

The population was estimated at 11.0 million in 2011 and its life expectancy at birth was 48.7 years. Its religion is 53 per cent Muslim, 20 per cent Catholic, 14 per cent Protestant, 7 per cent animist and a few atheists and other religions. In the year 2011 the birth rate was 38.7 per 1,000 and the death rate 15.2. This gives a rate of natural increase of 2.4 per cent. It is situated in Central Africa south of Libya. In 2011 the average woman had 4.9 children (CIA 2012, p. 143).

The whole area of childbirth is problematical for the country. It has one of the highest maternal mortality rates in the world with a lifetime risk of one in fourteen suffering a maternal death. Less than one in five maternities are attended by a skilled practitioner.

The country has very low usage of contraception with less than one in twenty women of childbearing age using it in 2010. Despite there being a low demand for contraception, only 12 per cent of the demand was met.

Observers report that, although abortion is illegal except to protect the woman's life or health, it is rarely prosecuted. There has been a problem of rape with an estimated about one in twenty of these leading to an unwanted pregnancy (FetterKa 2012).

Congo-Democratic Republic (DR)

The population was estimated at 73.6 million in 2012. Its religion is 50 per cent Catholic, 20 per cent Protestant, 10 per cent Kimbanguist, 10 per cent Muslim and 10 per cent other (CIA 2012, p. 166). In the year 2011 the birth rate was 37.1 per 1,000 and the death rate 10.8. This gives a rate of natural increase of 2.6 per cent. In 2011 the average woman had 5.1 children (CIA 2012, p. 166). The capital city is Kinshasa with a population of 8.4 million in 2009 (CIA 2012, p. 166).

The country endured a brutal civil war during which an estimated three to five million people were killed as the country became a battleground for the armies of seven different countries (Martins 2004, CIA 2012, p. 167). Improvements began in 2002 with the departure of many foreign troops.

Human Rights Watch (2005) said that women in Eastern Congo have suffered tremendous sexual violence. Victims are aged between 4 months to 84 years. The war situation has resulted in many soldiers committing terrible acts of rape and mutilation of women. There are drugs which can protect against HIV/AIDS if taken up to 72 hours after an assault, but few women take them. An unmarried girl who has been raped has little chance of marriage. If the pregnancy continues the baby is often rejected by the girl. One commented before the birth 'what if my baby looks like my rapist'. Pratt and Werchickl reported that one of the problems was that many soldiers believe that sex with a prepubescent or post-menopausal woman can give strength and protect from injury and death. One young women was interviewed and said

> The attack happened at night and we were forced to flee into the bush … four men took me. They all raped me. At the time I was nine months pregnant. They gang raped me and pushed sticks up my vagina – that's when my baby died – they said it was better than killing me. (Martens 2004)

She continued to say that her community shuns her and now all she wishes to do is to get well. A later study interviewed 4,000 women over a four year period and found that over 60 per cent of rapes were by armed men and half occurred in the victims' homes. More recently there has been a change. In 2004, only one per cent of rapes were by civilians but in 2008 it had risen to over a third (Ross 2010). The latest evidence available indicates that rape is still a problem in Congo DR.

We have seen that the data for the period 2005–2010 showed that the contraceptive prevalence rate in Congo DR was 18 per cent which is well below the world average of 63.0 per cent, An investigation by Kistof and colleagues into contraception in Congo DR reported 'We chatted with families whose huts were overflowing with small children – who the parent couldn't afford to educate, feed or protect from diseases' (2010).

Some of the respondents said that they wanted many children in the expectation that some would die. Finance can also be a problem. One woman had eight children two of whom had died. She was happy to stop reproducing but said that she could not afford the one dollar a month that the hospital charges for contraception.

Kistof's report quoted 'Emily' who was 25 years old who said 'I did not want to get pregnant. I was afraid – I never heard of birth control.' There was not only ignorance but there were also restrictions. All the clinics they visited had a precondition that they would only sell contraceptives to women if they brought their husbands with them to prove he agreed. Kistof commented that the pill has been around for over 50 years but still it has not reached parts of Africa (2010).

Abortion is legal only when the pregnancy threatens the woman's life or the foetus suffers from abnormalities. Clearly there is much to be done to seek a peaceful environment where people can be safe and making their own choices about their lifestyle.

Côte D'Ivoire

The country has had close ties to France since gaining its independence in 1960. However, it suffered civil wars and there is still a great amount of tension leading to the presence of thousands of UN peacekeepers. Its population was 22.0 million in 2012 and growth of population has been 2.2 per cent per annum. Its birth rate in 30.4 per thousand and death rate 10.0. Its largest city and the seat of Government is Abidjan with a population of 4.0 million. Its religion is two in five (39 per cent) Muslim, one third (33 per cent) Christian, 12 per cent indigenous beliefs and 17 per cent none. Its life expectancy at birth is 57.3 years and the average woman has 3.8 children (CIA 2012, p. 180).

A law of 1981 was anti-abortion except to save the woman's life with penalty being up to five years in prison and fines. There are many unsafe abortions in the country. Sixteen-year-old Korotoumoul Bakayoko was three months pregnant and thought she would bring shame on her family. She inserted a tree bark into her vagina together with ground glass. She went to hospital but died. In part this was because there was not the requisite medical equipment. A study of 2,400 women found that abortion was very common with a 2005 study finding that over a third (34 per cent) of women reported having had one. It does seem that many operations were carried out safely in hospital despite the law. A study of young people aged between 13–24 years found that 70 per cent of their abortions were carried out safely. Sana Sanago commented on the situation:

> It would be better to legalize abortions, even if they are condemned by certain religions, so that they can take place under the required medical conditions, to avoid the death of young girls or women.

She continued to say that in the current situation many women having terminations became sterile (Ouattara 2005). There have been some positive developments on the contraceptive front, for example, the introduction of injectable hormones (Oumar 2012).

Egypt

The population was estimated at 83.7 million in 2011 and its life expectancy at birth was 72.9 years. Its religion is 90 per cent Muslim (mostly Sunni) and ten per cent Christian (mainly Coptic). In the year 2011 the birth rate was 24.2 per 1,000 and the death rate 4.8. This gives a rate of natural increase of 1.9 per cent. In 2011 the average woman had 2.9 children which is a 0.2 per cent reduction on 2005 (CIA 2012, p. 220).

Egypt was the first Arab country to adopt a national population policy. The government adopted a plan to reduce fertility in 1962 and established the Supreme Council for Population and Family Planning in 1965. In 1981 Egypt became the first Arab country to ratify the convention to eliminate all forms of discrimination against women. In 1994 Cairo was the venue for the important. International Conference on Population and Development. The Egyptian Family Planning Association, started providing reproductive health services countrywide in 1995. Contraceptive use increased from (41 per cent) married and cohabiting women in 1990 to 60 per cent in 2005–2010. This is just below the world average of 63 per cent and is high in comparison to other countries in the area. However, it remains the case that 14 per cent of births were reported as unwanted and if contraception had been used the birth rate would have fallen from just under three children per women to 2.4.

IPPF reported in 2007 that it had 139 clinics all over the country. The efforts of the Member Association to combat unsafe abortion focused on encouraging men and women to use contraceptive methods in order to prevent unwanted pregnancies. In part this is by use of mobile clinics.

In 1993 the maternal mortality ratio was 170 per 100,000 and unsafe abortion deaths were a significant contributing factor. In 2008 the maternal mortality ratio decreased to 82/100,000. So it had declined by over a half in 15 years and more reductions are expected (CIA 2012, p. 220).

Abortion in Egypt has a long history, in fact, one of the earliest known descriptions of abortion appears in an Egyptian medical text. A female inserted a plant covered in honey and dates into her vagina (Cunningham 2013). Recently an article entitled 'Abortion is illegal and common in Egypt' reported that a study of country areas found that amongst unwanted pregnancies in rural areas 31 per cent were successfully aborted and a further 21 per cent were failed attempts (El Damanhoury).

One of the problems within an Egyptian context is that if a woman has apparently blackened the family name she might suffer an 'honour killing' which the perpetrators would think has 'washing away their disgrace'. One observer told of 22-year-old Amira who went through a clandestine abortion to escape severe retribution. She was in love with her boyfriend of five years and commented:

> I couldn't tell my friends because they would judge me a as a sinner and would never speak to me again, if they said anything to my family I could be killed.

For the operation she told the doctor she was married but could not afford to bring up a child. There was a slight liberalization of the law in on March 2010. The Health committee of the People's Assembly extended the law to include provision for a woman to have an abortion for the benefit of her health. It was opposed by the Muslim hierarchy who said that abortion 'intervened in God's will.

If the law stays restrictive then it seems that there will be an extension of abortion by drugs. Dubliette reports that if women go on the website http//www.women on web.org/ they will be able to obtain abortifacient drugs (2013).

Ethiopia

The population was estimated at 92.8 million in 2012 which is the thirteenth largest in the world. Its life expectancy at birth was 56.6 years in 2011. Its religion is 44 per cent Ethiopian Orthodox, 34 per cent Muslim, 19 per cent Protestant and three per cent traditional. In the year 2011 the birth rate was 42.6 per 1,000 and the death rate 10.8. This gives a rate of natural increase of 3.2 per cent which is an increase from a figure of 2.0 quoted for 2003 and is the fifth fastest growth rate in the world (CIA 2012, p. 238), Wright 2006, p. 486). In 2011 the average woman had 6.0 children. Its capital city is Addis Ababa with a population estimated in 2009 at 2.9 million people (CIA 2012, p. 238).

The Guttmacher Institute states the use of contraceptives is 57 per cent amongst married couples in Addis Ababa which is much higher than Ethiopia as a whole where it is 14 per cent (2010). The low levels of contraceptive use in 2008 led to over two in five (42 per cent) of pregnancies being unintended. In 2005, one in three Ethiopian women of childbearing age (15–44) had an unmet need for contraception in that they were able to become pregnant, did not want a child soon or at all and were not using a method of contraception. In the years 2005–2010 only 15 per cent of women of childbearing age were using contraception. There is clearly a large, unmet need. (World Bank 2012).

In 2004 in order to reduce the harm caused by illegal abortion and to conform to international human rights treaties, Ethiopia expanded the circumstances under which abortion is permitted to include the pregnant woman's lack of capacity to care for a child because of her age or physical or mental health. Minors automatically fall under this provision. Prior to 2004, abortion was permitted only to save a woman's life or protect her physical health and in cases of rape, incest or serious foetal impairment. Ministry of Health guidelines now prescribe 'Woman centered care', that is,

> a comprehensive approach to providing abortion services that takes account the various factors that influence a woman's individual mental and physical health needs, her personal circumstances, and her ability to access services.

The guidelines also provide that abortions should be provided within three days of a woman's request, that proof of rape or incest is not required for abortions on those grounds, and that a minor is not requited to present proof of age (Center for Reproductive Rights 2005).

The Guttmacher Institute commented, however, 'Notwithstanding the new law almost six out of ten abortions in Ethiopia are unsafe' (2010). Its data for 2008 indicated that an estimated 328,500 induced abortions were performed for an annual rate of 23 abortions per 1,000 women aged 15–44. The average age of women having abortions was 23 years and the majority (53 per cent) were single. One of its findings is that urban areas have a higher abortion rate than the rest of the country. In Addis Ababa, it is 46 per 1,000 women (15–44) which is more than double the national average. A discussion of the reasons for this will occur at the end of the chapter.

Researchers report a high number of women suffer from adverse complications from abortion and four out of ten women seeking post abortion show signs of infection or invasive injuries. However, care has improved since guidelines were introduced in 2006 (Guttmacher Institute 2010).

Ghana

The population was estimated at 25.2 million (2012). Its life expectancy at birth was 61.4 years in 2011 and the population growth rate was 1.8 per cent per annum. The birth rate was 27.0 per 1,000 population and the death rate was 8.6. According to the 2,000 census its religion is 54 per cent Protestant, 15 per cent Catholic, 16 per cent Muslim, nine per cent traditional and six per cent none. Its capital is Accra with a population of 2.7 million (2009).

Ghana was one of the first countries in sub-Saharan Africa to adopt a population policy and it aimed to reduce population growth in order to aid socio-economic development. The following May the Ghanaian National Family Planning programme was launched (Gyimah 2011). In 1994 the National Policy Council aimed to reduce the total fertility rate from 6.0 births per woman to 4.0 in 2010 and 3.0 in 2020. In the event it more than matched the target. The rate had dropped to 3.8 in 2008 and 3.4 in 2011 (Gyimah 2011, CIA 2012, p. 283).

In 1985 the abortion law was liberalized to allow it in cases where women faced problems of physical or mental health, for rape or incest or in the case of foetal abnormality. In 2006 the Ministry of Health and the Ghanaian Health Service developed a protocol designed to lead to the safe provision of abortion (Asami 2013). Many women are not aware that abortion can be legal in this range of circumstances and a survey found that only four per cent could identify the grounds for which abortion is legal.

This lack of knowledge was one factor leading women to seek unsafe terminations. One woman with an unwanted pregnancy was called Naa (she wished to keep her family name a secret). She was 20 years old and told how at the age of 15 years she had become pregnant. She was the eldest child and wanted to get a good job so she could look after her mother and sister. She was worried that if her school found out she was pregnant it would expel her which would reduce her employment opportunities. She obtained a bitter herbal concoction from friends and after she had taken it began bleeding. After an hour her mother came home from work earlier than expected which was fortunate as she was able to take Naa to the hospital where the doctor gave her an abortion which saved her life. In this matter she fared better than one young girl who arrived at a hospital after an abortion and was not treated but allowed to bleed to death (Asami 2013).

Other young women use a variety of methods to try and procure an abortion. One mentioned as being use in Ghana was a chorkor bomb which is placed inside the vagina. One commentator stated 'When the bomb explodes, it tears open the vagina' (Asami 2013).

Some doctors take a view that the law should be extended but face some difficulties. Dr Otu-Nyarko commented:

> If you come out and say that abortion is legal and that the woman has a right over her own body and the right to say what is good or bad for her, you are stigmatized. (Asami 2013)

MSI, PI and Ipas Ghana are all active in the country and have an educational and clinical role to play. In December 2012 Ipas Ghana arranged a meeting at which its leader Dr Koma S. Jehu-Appiah stated:

> The women are dying and we are doing nothing about it. We are talking about it because we do not want the women to die. Refusing women access to comprehensive abortion care services leads them to quack doctors. (Asami 2013)

Biney said research into unwanted pregnancies leading to abortion indicated that from 2002–2007 three out of ten (28 per cent) were due to contraceptive failure and seven out of ten (70 per cent) were due to non-use. She analysed some of the reasons for non-use and found that some women had a lack of information, others stopped using contraception because of health problems and a number of women reported that they were raped by their partner. One comparative figure Biney reported was that amongst women of the developed world if they found they had an unwanted pregnancy then over seven out of ten (73 per cent) would have an abortion whereas in the developing world it was only just over half (54 per cent) (Asami 2013).

Guinea

The country gained independence from France in 1958 and has had a checkered history with military rule and election irregularities. The first free election was held in 2010 (CIA 2012, p. 308). Its population was estimated at 10.9 million in 2011 with a increase of 2.6 per cent per annum and life expectancy at birth of 58.6 years. The average woman has 5.0 children and its birth rate is 36.6 per 1,000 and death rate 10.2 (2011). Its religion is 85 per cent Muslim, eight per cent Christian and seven per cent indigenous beliefs. The capital city is Conakry with a population of 1.6 million (2009) (CIA 2012, p. 309). The UN reported that in 2000 only one in ten women were using modern forms of contraception and under half a per cent were using condoms. However, things have developed. Bayer Health Care has been providing long term contraception under the trade name of Jadelle at a cut price rate. It reduced a commercial price of $18 to $8.50. A young mother called 'Mercy' was one of those to benefit. She had her fifth child when she missed a pill and was happy that the injectable would give her some respite from continual childbearing (Issak 2013).

The law was slightly liberalized in 1991. It allowed abortion to protect the woman's physical and mental health. However, it was still relatively restrictive (Issak 2013). It was one of the countries targeted by Women on Waves AKA Women on the Web. Its publicity states: 'Living in a country where safe abortion is not available? Get abortion pills online.'

Kenya

The population was estimated at 43.0 million in 2012. In 2011 its life expectancy at birth was 63.1 years. Its religion is 45 per cent Protestant, 33 per cent Catholic, 10 per cent Muslim, and 10 per cent indigenous beliefs. In the year 2011 the birth rate was 32 per 1,000 and the death rate 7.3. This gives a rate of natural increase of 2.4 per cent. In the later 1960s and 1970s the average woman had over eight children. By 2005 the average woman had 5.0 children and in 2011 it was 4.0 (Wright 2006, p. 482; CIA 2012, p. 388). Its capital city is Nairobi with an estimated population of 3.4 million in 2009 (CIA 2012, p. 387).

A study in 2009 found that a quarter of married women had an unmet need for contraception in that they did not want to become pregnant but had no method in place. Shahnaz Sharif, director of public health told IRIN:

> We provide contraception free in government facilities and we create a lot of media campaigns around the issue ... (however) ... cultural and religious beliefs at times might hamper a wider uptake of contraception. (2012)

She continued to say that sex education in schools had proved controversial but they had done their best to keep everyone on board. In the Introduction I mentioned the 2012 conference in London on contraception especially in poorer countries. Wycliffe Oparanya represented Kenya and the country signed up to help promote Family Planning. A study of the method of contraception in 2008 showed that almost half (47.5 per cent) of the women had injectables. A further 16 per cent were on the pill. Male methods were rarely used with only four per cent of couples using the condom and vasectomy was below one per cent. There may well be a case for further activity in male responsibility (USAID 2012).

The 2010 new constitution for Kenya explicitly legalizes abortion on extended grounds. However, the GI states that the language is such that some possible providers might feel inhibited to carry out terminations (Hussein 2012). Peggy, whose boyfriend abandoned her told IRIN: 'We have a clinic here in Dandora where an old lady helps many women have abortions. I bled for two days nonstop'. She continued to say that her mother took her to the hospital where she had a blood transfusion and other treatment that saved her life. She said that she was suspicious of contraception. Some people said that it made one fat and others that it made one thin. Others said it caused sterility (IRIN 2012).

One of the few studies of abortion was conducted by the Ministry of Health in 2004. This estimated that there were 300,000 abortions each year and that 20,000 women were hospitalized (IRIN 2012). The Ministry of Health reported that in 2012 there were 465,000 abortions and that the vast majority were unsafe. Over a quarter of the women (120,000) sought medical treatment for abortion complications. The rate of abortions was 48 per 1,000 women 15–45 which is higher than nearly every country in Africa (International Campaign 2013a).

Madagascar

The population was estimated at 22.6 million in 2011 and its life expectancy at birth was 64 years. Its religion is 52 per cent indigenous beliefs, 41 per cent Christian and seven per cent Muslim (Wright 2006, p. 625). In the year 2011 the birth rate was 37.1 per 1,000 and the death rate 7.6. The rate of natural increase was 3.0 per cent. In 2011 the average woman had 5.0 children (CIA 2012, p. 448).

We have seen that the French had passed an act proscribing contraception in 1920 with a provision for acceptance for women with health problems. At least until 2013 this was still in prospect. Nevertheless, from 1967 organizations linked to the IPPF began playing an active role in promotion of contraception and the Government took a more active role. In 2011 the UN drew attention to the fact that the country had a 'striking success' in improving family planning and reproductive health. The use of modern contraceptives had tripled over a ten year period. It rose from 9.7 per cent in 1997 to 29.2 per cent in 2008–9. In making this change it overtook the Government's ambitious goal of 28 per cent by 2009. This change was made despite the country's high rate of poverty and a rural population leading to transport difficulties. It was achieved by a variety of agencies working together. They provided sufficient equipment and it was very important that they had the support of the Government.

MSI began working in the country in 1992 and by 2013 was offering a full range of sexual and Reproductive Health information across the country with 14 clinics and 15 outreach teams which aimed to provide long acting contraception (MSI 2013a).

Although abortion is still officially illegal except to save the life of the woman an estimate by a local organization was that around 24 per cent of women had had one.

Malawi

The population of Malawi was estimated at 16.2 million in 2012. In 2011, life expectancy at birth was 52.3 years. The religion is 83 per cent Christian, 13 per cent Muslim and four per cent other or none (CIA 2012, p.452). In the year 2011 the birth rate was 40.4 per 1,000 and the death rate was 12.8.

The country became independent in 1964. Bakil Muluzi was in office from 1994 to 2004. He introduced far more open government and, for example, disclosed that his brother had died of HIV/AIDS. In 2004 a programme of action to combat HIV was introduced. Still in 2009 the adult prevalence was over one in ten (11 per cent) adults (CIA 2012, p. 452).

In 2013 the BBC reported that since 2007 there has been real progress towards economic growth and that the subsidy of fertilizers had boosted output. However, it also commented that rapid population growth has meant that an increase in production was needed to try and keep level. In 2011 the increase in population was 2.8 per cent and the average woman had 5.4 children – well over double the rate to maintain a stable population (CIA 2012, p. 453).

There have been efforts to tackle the problem of overpopulation. In 2000 the Malawi Demographic and Health Survey made some important findings. One was that 64 per cent of non-pregnant women who did not want children were nevertheless not using modern contraception. It did however, find that Depo-Provera had increased in usage from one per cent in 1992 to six per cent in 1996 and 16 per cent in 2000. This increase continued so that 27 per cent of women were using injectables in 2010. The overall increase in modern contraception was from 28 per cent in 2000 to 42 per cent in 2010. In 2012 the Vice President Khumbo Kachale promised to raise contraceptive prevalence to 60 per cent by 2020 and that there would be special efforts to ensure that teenagers did not get pregnant before adulthood. He recognized that would be a necessity for increased resources to be available (*Nyasa Times* 2012).

The gaps in contraceptive care led to a number of unwanted pregnancies. In 2009 a study by the Malawi Ministry of Health and the US-based organization IPAS, estimated that there were 70,000 unsafe abortions each year and that these were the cause of 17 per cent of maternal deaths. Kanyalika calculated that on an average day there were 12–16 maternal deaths and three or four deaths from unsafe abortion. She called for the government to find better ways of helping women (2013).

Seode White, an activist, commented that the poor could not afford a safe abortion and some of them suffered sterility as a consequence. Therefore, 'It is high time Malawi takes a leaf from other African countries like Zambia and South Africa where abortion is legal'. There has been some concerted action on this front. In March 2013 the Gender, Children and Social Welfare minister Anita Kalinde, tabled the Gender Equality Bill which would allow women to have the right to choose to have a child without coercion or duress. It was unanimously voted for in Parliament, but has not passed into law as of May 2013.

The Catholic Church made clear its opposition to contraception and abortion in a pastoral letter (*Nyasa Times* 2013). It said 'At stake is an effort to break the traditional link between sexual intercourse and procreation'. The *Nyasa Times* (2 March 2013) reported:

> Against the argument that the woman has a right to her own body and, therefore, she can decide what to do with the foetus, the bishops say it must be asserted that the right of the unborn to life takes precedence over the right of the woman to control her body.

I have pointed out that Catholics in the West used to believe that a woman's life should be sacrificed rather than an abortion occur. It seems that bishops are returning to this harsh position. The bishops also denounced homosexuality as threatening to the existence of marriage (*Nyasa Times* 2013).

A different approach was taken by Pastor Mangom, a Presbyterian who said 'The Government should consider legalizing abortion so as to reduce death rates'. Clearly at the moment the jury is out as to whether abortion will be legalized

Mali

The population of Mali was estimated at 14.5 million in 2011 and life expectancy was 53.1 years. The average woman has 6.4 children which is the third highest in the world. The infant mortality rate is also the third highest in the world. Three in ten of its children under five are underweight (28 per cent 2006). Its religion is 90 per cent Muslim and nine per cent indigenous beliefs. Just under half (46 per cent) of the population were literate in 2003 although this will be expected to improve as male children had nine years' schooling and females seven years in 2009 (CIA, p. 463).

The government has been promoting contraception. In 1972 Mali became the first Francophone country to repeal the 1920 Act placing restrictions on birth control. In 1991 a population policy was officially adopted. Its goal is to increase contraceptive usage to 60 per cent of the population by 2020. This it hopes will help reduce the number of its abortions as the Government sees a major cause of it to be the unmet need for contraception (UN 2013a). During the period 2005–2010 less than one in ten (8 per cent) of fertile women (15–49) were using contraception which is one of the lowest rates in the world.

Morocco

The population was estimated at 32.3 million in 2011 and life expectancy at birth was 76.1 years. The religion is just under 99 per cent Muslim, one per cent Christian and around 6,000 Jewish people (CIA 2012, p. 500). In the year 2011 the birth rate was 19.0 per 1,000 and the death rate 4.8. In 2011 the average woman had 2.2 children (CIA 2012, p. 500).

A French law of 10 July 1939 prohibited the advertisement and sale of contraceptives. The Government of Morocco has supported family planning since independence in 1956 and has recognized the influence of demographic factors on the national debate. Contraceptives have been distributed free of charge in government family planning centres. Beginning with the development plan of 1968–1972, population issues, including family planning, have been accorded high priority in the planning process in Morocco (UN 2004, p. 57).

Morocco's abortion law was first liberalized in 1967. At that time, Article 453 of the Penal Code was amended by Royal Decree (1 July) to provide that the performance of an abortion would not be punished when it was a necessary measure to safeguard the physical health of the woman and is openly performed by a physician or a surgeon with the consent of the spouse. If there is no husband or the husband refuses or is prevented from giving his consent, the physician or surgeon may not perform the abortion without the written opinion of the chief medical officer of the province or prefecture, certifying that the intervention is the only means of safeguarding the health of the woman. If the physician believes that the woman's life is in jeopardy, the consent of the spouse or opinion of the chief medical officer is not required. The physician or surgeon must however, give his opinion to the chief medical officer of the province or prefecture.

In all other cases abortion is illegal under the Penal Code, although some evidence exists that foetal impairment may be taken into account under medical indications. Local IPPF commentators suggest that despite the law illegal abortion appears to be quite widespread in Morocco with many women resorting to it as a contraceptive method. In addition, it appears that the incidence of illegal abortion is underestimated. Many women obtaining an illegal abortion appear to be married women from the urban upper and middle classes who undergo the procedure in a private clinic. Surveys of public hospitals suggest that a significant number of admissions are of women from the lower socio-economic groups suffering from complications of septic abortion.

Mozambique

The population was estimated at 23.5 million in 2012. In 2011 its life expectancy at birth was 52.0 years. Its religion is 28 per cent Catholic, 28 per cent Protestant, 18 per cent Muslim, seven per cent other and 19 per cent none (CIA 2012). In the year 2011 the birth rate was 39 per 1,000 and the death rate 12.8. In 2011 the rate of natural increase was 2.4 per cent and the average woman had 5.4 children (CIA 2012, p. 504). Its capital city is Maputo with a population of 1.6 million (2009).

Contraceptive use is very low. The United Nations stated in 1999 that it was used by 7.3 per cent (UN 2004). Abortion has a quasi-legal status. Although strictly allowed only for the woman's life or health, a 1981 Ministry of Health decree supported a broad interpretation of this risk. Consequently, abortion on request has been available in several public hospitals ever since (Gallo et al. 2004). Most of these abortions are performed by using misoprostol followed by manual vacuum aspiration 24 hours later. The cost of the abortion in 2002 was about $15 US which is a substantial sum in a country where 78 per cent of the population were known to live on less than $2 a day.

Gallo reported one in seven women die during pregnancy, although such a high figure is difficult to believe (2004). Nevertheless, deaths which do occur are in large part related to unsafe abortions. In 1995 a study conducted in Maputo Central Hospital found that women attending for complications tended to be the younger and poorer women. Four out of five said that they did not know of the possibility of hospital based abortions. Others had difficulty with the large amount of information needed by hospitals.

In 2002 the Ministry of Health conducted an assessment of abortion services to inform efforts to make abortion safer. The study surveyed 461 women in 37 public hospitals and four health centres who were facing abortion-related complications. In addition 128 providers were interviewed. The results showed that the patients had to face a lengthy waiting time in order to secure treatment. Fewer women were receiving pain relief than providers thought were usual and less than half the women received follow up care information. Of those women who wanted to avoid pregnancy only 27 per cent said that they had received a contraceptive method. The results of the survey led to the Ministry trying to improve training of providers (Gallo et al. 2004).

Niger

The country gained its independence from France in 1960. It is one of the poorest countries in the world and in 2009 ranked 174 out of 178 countries on the Human Development Index (Potts et al. 2011). Only 12 per cent of Niger's land receives enough rain to sustain agriculture and the soil is low in nutrients, over grazed and losing topsoil. Poor harvests in 2010 let to the need for the World Food Programme providing emergency food aid to five million people and in that year 44 per cent of children suffered from chronic malnutrition and a high proportion of these could face a life with growth stunted by poor diet (Potts et al. 2011).

The country has suffered a number of military coups and periods of extended drought. In 2011 its population was 17.1 million and its increase 3.6 per cent per annum. Its birth rate is the highest in the world at 50.6 per 1,000 population and death rate 13.8. The median age of marriage amongst women is 15.5 years and the average woman has 7.2 children. It is the only country where the average number of births is over seven (CIA 2011, Potts et al. 2011). One in four women over the age of 40 has ten or more children and a study in 2006 found that the average man wanted 12.6 children (Potts et al. 2011). Depending on future birth rates the UN estimates that the population will rise to between 47 million and 59 million in 2050 leading to Potts and colleagues remark on the urgent need to slow population growth (Potts et al. 2011).

Its religion is 80 per cent Muslim and 20 per cent Christian or indigenous beliefs. The capital city is Niamey with 1.0 million people (CIA 2012, p. 531). In 2007 only 15 per cent of women had any primary education and only one per cent had completed primary school.

The country has provided free contraception since 2002 which it has promoted by radio broadcasts. However, by 2009 only 11 per cent of married Niger women aged 15–49 were practising contraception and only five per cent were using modern methods – mainly the pill or the IUD. The most common reasons given for non-use of contraception were 'desire for more children', 'menopause' and 'sterility'. Although the demand for contraception is generally low, nevertheless in Niger only 42 per cent of the demand is met. Furthermore, one positive factor is that the desired family size is a 'moving target' and will decline as people see the benefit of better health and nutrition. Potts et al., state that after decades of inaction any policy which simply advocated contraception was likely to be problematical as the lack of health infrastructure and shortages of personnel would restrict what could be done. Some women will still use traditional methods such as lactational amenorrhoea and therefore it is important not to permit artificial feeding (Potts et al. 2011).

Despite the generally pro-natalist environment, one in six women report having an unwanted pregnancy.

Nigeria

The population was estimated at 170.1 million in 2012 and its life expectancy at birth was 52.1 years. Its religion is around 50 per cent Muslim, 40 per cent Christian and 10 per cent indigenous beliefs. In the year 2011 the birth rate was 39.2 per 1,000 and the death rate 13.5. The rate of natural increase was 2.6 and the average woman had 5.4 children (CIA 2012, p. 534). Although Lagos with 10.2 million people is the largest city, the capital is Abuja with a population of 1.9 million (2009) (CIA 2012, p. 534).

There used to be a strong prejudice against contraception in Nigeria with the subject being taboo and the users 'sinners' especially in the mainly Muslim north. In 2008 only 2.7 per cent of married women in the north-west states and four per cent in the north-east states were using contraception and it was only a one in ten (10 per cent) average for the country as a whole. However, things have been changing. Agatha Lawson commented she was 'having long discussions with religious and traditional leaders working to raise awareness'. Similar evidence is provided by Alhaji Sani Umar who said he passed on information through traditional and religious leaders using community meetings. There are also radio and television programmes which carry information about contraception. Over four out of five (84 per cent) have heard of family planning by these, although only 57 per cent have tried the methods themselves (IRIN 2011).

There has been some opposition. In 2008 the south-western state of Anambra banned condoms, although Lawson said that the authorities did not interfere with her work. Furthermore, in April 2011 the Government set aside $3 million in order to provide free contraception in hospitals. Methods included condoms, intra-uterine devices and long-acting implants /(IRIN 2011).

In 1996–1997 Henshaw and colleagues estimated that there were 610,000 abortions in Nigeria each year for a rate 25 per 1,000 women aged 15–44 (Henshaw et al. 1998). This is higher than a 1980 estimate of a Government Committee of Enquiry of 500,000 illegal abortions (Population Division 2007a). This survey, which was based on a study of 672 facilities, found that 27 per cent of private physicians and fifteen per cent of public facilities performed abortions about equally by dilation and curettage and manual vacuum aspiration. There are many providers available, Abortions can be obtained from physicians at a modest cost, but nevertheless, many women prefer the convenience, privacy and lower cost of non-physicians or pharmacists. An estimate from the Guttmacher Institute published in 2008 calculated that the number of abortions had increased to 750,000 a year of which around 60 per cent (456,000) were deemed to be unsafe (Walker 2008).

These abortions are carried despite the fact that they are largely illegal. Two laws apply to the country. In the largely Muslim north the law is the Penal Code of 1959, while in the south the Criminal Code of 1916 is in effect. This second law is based on the British 1861 Act, which has been interpreted liberally in at least one case along the lines of the British 1938 Bourne decision to include wider grounds, including rape.

There are high number of deaths from abortion which in part may be due to the fact that an estimated 26 per cent of women with complications do not seek medical help (Grimes et al. 2006). One such death was that of Gloria Oguntola who bled to death and whose father John was quoted as saying 'We do not know who to hold responsible because she could not tell us before she died' (Olori 2007). Other women suffer long term health consequences. Toyin Aje became pregnant but her boyfriend told her he would not help to raise the child. She proposed to seek an abortion but was unable to get one in a public hospital. She sought help from a man who worked in a pharmacy in Abuja. He was neither a doctor nor a pharmacist but sold her drugs. She was five months pregnant and the foetus died and was left in her womb. She began to experience severe pain and was eventually treated in hospital. Although they were able to save her life she was told that she would be sterile (Olori 2007). Such incidents are very common and overall only 40 per cent of Nigerian abortions are estimated as being carried out by doctors.

One of the reasons why abortions have been particularly unsafe in the past is that the methods use have been very dangerous. Walker states that one method used was to use a sharp stick to break the amniotic sac. Another was to use a toxic mixture of fiercely hot alligator chili peppers and chemicals such as alum which they would ingest into their bodies (Walker 2012).

In 1982 an attempt to liberalize the law was sponsored by the Society of Gynaecologists and Obstetricians of Nigeria. This would have allowed abortion on the grounds that two physicians agreed 'there were substantial risk to the life of a pregnant woman, or injury to her physical and mental health or to any existing children in her family greater than if the pregnancy were terminated'. There would have been exceptions for conscience and the potential law bears strong overtones of the debate at the time of the British 1967 Act. However, the change was opposed by religious groups and by the Nigerian National Council of Women's Societies and failed (Population Division 2007a).

The Government showed its concern about population when in 1988 its set up a National Population Policy which encourages family planning. However, progress toward modern forms of contraception has been slower than most would like.

The case for a new law and more liberal practice remains strong. In 1991 the Federal Ministry of Health called for a change in the law (Henshaw et al. 1998).

Boniface Oye-Adenirian, the President of the African Medical Association and an obstetrician and gynaecologist in Lagos commented:

> For us to reduce the carnage to our women through unsafe abortions, the law has to regulate abortion services, determine who performs it and where it can be performed. If abortion services become more available in public hospitals quacks will be discouraged. (*International Press News* 2007)

There is a very strong case for increasing the availability of safe operations.

Rwanda

In 1959, three years before the country gained its independence from Belgium the majority group, Hutus, overthrew the Tutsi king and over the next few years thousands of Tutsis were killed or driven into exile. Further violence led to genocide against Tutsis and Rwandans killed up to a million of their own citizens. More peaceful developments led to the country joining the Commonwealth in 2009. The population size in 2011 was 11.7 million and growth each year was 2.8 per cent. The population growth is a source of concern for many observers as Rwanda is over ten times as densely populated as the average for sub-Saharan Africa. It has 355 people per square kilometre compared to the average of 32 (Solo 2008). Its life expectancy at birth is 58.4 years. The average woman has 4.8 children and the birth rate is 36.1 per 1,000. The death rate is 9.6. Its religion is 57 per cent Catholic 37 per cent Protestant (including Adventists) and five per cent Muslim The capital is Kigali with a population approaching a million (CIA 2012, p. 603).

Despite the high Catholic population President Kagame said that Family planning is a national priority. Genocide disrupted the development of modern contraception. So in 1992, 13 per cent were using modern contraception. The percentage languished at 4 per cent. It subsequently rose to 10 per cent in 2005 and 27 per cent in 2008 (Solo 2008). Further rises are to be expected.

In discussing the benefits of contraception Umulesi (2012) commented that by spreading contraception inroads could be make into curbing the number of abortions which he estimated at 60,000 a year. He stated that the Guttmacher Institute estimated an abortion rate of 25 per women aged 15–44. In 2012 Rwanda had a new law decriminalizing abortion in some circumstances. In the revised penal code abortion is legalized when the pregnancy is a result of rape, forced marriage or sexual intercourse with a close family member. In addition it decriminalizes abortion when the pregnancy jeopardizes the health of the woman or that of the foetus (Bumwe 2012). Government officials said that changes in society necessitated a revised abortion law. Jacqueline Bakamur said the previous law was outmoded, 'it was dated 1977 and therefore was not matching the current situation in Rwanda. It is modernizing it according to the development of the country.' Others made the claim that the new law would reduce the number of clandestine abortions that are likely to be unsafe (Bumwe 2012). Of course such a minor liberalization will only help to legalize a small proportion of abortions in the country.

The Centre for Reproductive Health welcomed the change in law (2012) and also the fact that the Government supports the Maputo Protocol.

Senegal

The country gained its independence from France in 1959 (joined at the time to French Sudan). Despite some political upheavals it has been one of Africa's most stable democracies. The population size in 2011 was 13.0 million and growth each year 2.5 per cent. Life expectancy at birth was 60.2 years in 2009. The average woman has 4.7 children and the birth rate is 36.2 per 1,000. The death rate is 9.1. The religion is 94 per cent Muslim, five per cent Christian. Dakar, the capital has a population of 2.8 million (2009).

The Government of Senegal is pressing for action on contraception, although there have been reports that there are shortage of supplies. One study in 2012 stated that implants were out of stock for 83 per cent of the year and injectables for 42 per cent of the time. However, they had started using the delivery drivers to report back on potential shortages.

Abortion is illegal except to save a woman's life but unsafe abortion has been reported as being common. 'You can't imagine the number of abortions that take place in Daka' said one gynaecologist 'every day dozens upon dozens'. He continued to say that he charged the equivalent to $375 for an abortion. This amount is over ten times the monthly salary of a servant (Karafin 2008). For those not able to pay these prices an article in *Ms* magazine stated:

> For the poor, the procedure usually entails dangerous do-it-yourself experiments. Women drink teas of boiled coins, seek injection of drugs such as acetate and oxytocin, and prepare cocktails of neem leaves and malaria drugs … . It would be difficult to overstate the gap between international charters and the reality on the ground in Dakar. (Karafin 2008)

Investigation by a Dutch radio station led to an abortionist in his 50s being interviewed in complete secrecy and anonymity. He had been performing abortions for over twenty years and commented that he regularly saw 'many young women':

> (I also) see company executives who want to conceal the pregnancy of their mistresses, mostly for social reasons. Sometimes I want to help friends or relatives who find themselves in a difficult position with their families because of an unplanned pregnancy. (Diagne 2012)

Two women reported very different experiences. Fatoumata told how she first went to a pharmacy and was directed to a certain doctor at a private clinic. There she was closely questioned to ensure that she would not cause any complications. She bargained over the price before agreeing to pay the equivalent of $120. It was a painful procedure which she said were the worse ten minutes of her life but she recovered.

An anonymous woman worked as a maid in Dakar. She says her boyfriend forced her to take pills and a drink concocted with a green powder. She delivered a foetus – she does not know whether it was alive. Her boyfriend took it away and buried it. She fell unconscious and her mother took her to the hospital. She was charged with infanticide and sentenced to two years imprisonment after which she was released.

The comments from gynaecologists and the experience of the two women suggests that it is the very much the rich who get the best treatment.

Somalia

The population of Somalia was estimated at 10.1 million in 2012. In 2011 its life expectancy at birth was 50.8 years. Its religion is almost completely Sunni Muslim (CIA 2012, p. 665). In the year 2011 the birth rate was 42.1 per 1,000 and the death rate 14.6. In 2011 the rate of natural increase was 1.6 and the average woman had 6.3 children which is the fourth highest in the world. The capital, Mogadishu, had a population of 1.4 million in 2009 (CIA 2012, p. 665).

Somalia gained independence from Britain and Italy in 1960. There was a brief period of democracy between 1960–69. However, especially in the 1980s there was a period of repression and in 1991 a period of anarchy and civil war until 1994. In 1993 a relief agency estimated that half of children under the age of five had died. Things improved and in 2012 Somalia adopted a new Constitution and gave more democratic rights and protected the right of women to have an abortion if her life was in danger. The celebration of these new freedoms was almost marred by two suicide bombers, although they were killed before they could do great damage (Pflanz 2012). The new constitution banned the practice of female circumcision which had caused many health problems including chronic pain.

The Government is concerned about the quality of maternal care and high levels of mortality. It is also worried about the morbidity and mortality due to unsafe abortion (UN 2013b). Only 14.5 per cent of women aged 15–49 years use contraception so an increase in availability could help reduce health problems (World Bank 2012).

South Africa

The population was estimated at 48.8 million in 2012. Four out of five are black African, one in ten white and nearly one in ten coloured. Its life expectancy at birth was 49.4 years and it is one of a few countries where men live longer than women.

Its religion is 80 per cent Christian of which seven per cent are Catholic. Only 1.5 per cent is Muslim and 15 per cent had no religion according to the 2001 census. In the year 2011 the birth rate was 19.3 per 1,000 and the death rate 17.2 which was the highest in the world.

In 2011 the average woman had 2.3 children and the population declined by 0.4 per cent. In 2009, 17.8 per cent of the adult population had the HIV/AIDS virus which is the fourth highest in the world (CIA 1012, p. 668). The largest city is Johannesburg with 3.6 million in 2009 and the capital is Pretoria.

Contraceptive use increased from half (51 per cent) married and cohabiting women in 1990 to (58 per cent) in the year 2,000 and nearly all of these were modern methods of contraception (UN 2004, p. 57)

The earlier policies on abortion were in part tied up with apartheid. Before 1975 abortion could be carried out under common law if there was a threat to 'a woman's well being'. The white political leadership was concerned that population changes were working against it. The Minister of Bantu Administration and Development M.C. Botha asked whites to have more children to ensure its continued existence as a Christian and Western country on the continent of Africa. Women were given tax advantages to encourage them in childbirth. In contrast, there were attempts to encourage the black population to use family planning. Consequently, the birth control became associated by some people with maintaining the apartheid regime. The Abortion and Sterilization Act was introduced in 1975 to restrict abortion. It allowed it only on the grounds of physical and mental health, sexual crimes such as rape and incest and foetal abnormality. The bureaucracy for obtaining an abortion was difficult. For example, the approval of two physicians was needed and neither of these was to be the one to perform the operation. Consequently there were few abortions carried out – around a thousand a year under the act (Guttmacher et al., 1998). Rich women could often obtain abortions by doctors performing a D&C in their office. However, this was risky as it was illegal. Other rich women could fly to London and many did so. However, poor women were reportedly using knitting needles or detergents or attending illegal and often unskilled practitioners (Guttmacher et al., 1998). In the period 1975–1996 there were an estimated 120,000 to 250,000 abortions a year. In 1994 the South African Medical Research Council carried out a study and found there were 45,000 hospital admissions and that over four hundred women had died. The cost of the hospitalization of women was calculated at $4.4 million.

The introduction of democracy led to a new law as the African National Congress (ANC) was in support and included it in its manifesto for the 1994 elections. The relevant statement was 'every woman must have the right to choose whether or not to have an early termination according to her own beliefs'. The law was passed by 209 votes to 87 on 11 December 1996 and came into effect on 1 February 1997. It granted abortion on request in the first twelve weeks of pregnancy and one commentator said that the law aimed to grant universal access to services for all women by giving them the sole right of consent (Hessini 2005). From 13–20 weeks abortion was allowed on more restricted grounds. It was permitted 'if a medical practitioner believes that the pregnancy threatens the mental or physical health of the woman or foetus' or in the case of rape and incest or if it 'affects the woman's socio-economic situation'. After 20 weeks abortion could be carried out in the case of severe foetal abnormality or in the case of the woman's life or health. The law was passed despite strong opposition of certain religious factions but with the support of women's groups and other health campaigners. One surprising feature of the law is that it permits abortion by nurse midwives who are trained and certified. Many abortions are now performed by nurses.

Legal abortion was a little slow to take off because of the reluctance of hospitals to provide the service and the small number of non-hospital providers. In 1997 there were only 34,000 recorded and 50,000 in 1998. These figures were well below the estimates for the number of illegal abortions before the act. The numbers then rose only slightly and were 59,000 in the year 2000. Then, presumably due to a decline in illegal abortions numbers began to rise more substantially to 90,000 in 2003 and 114,000 in 2004 (Johnston 2005).

South Sudan

Sudan was given its independence in 1956 and promised to give the South full participation in the political system. It reneged which led to a mutiny and to two periods of conflict over 50 years until a comprehensive peace agreement was signed in January 2005. It is estimated that 2.5 million died in the conflict. These were mostly civilians who died of starvation and drought (CIA 2012, p. 673).

South Sudan gained its independence in July 2011 and in 2012 the population was estimated at 10.6 million. Its religion is mainly Christian and animist (CIA 2012, p. 673). Its capital is Juba with a population estimated to be 250,000 in 2008 which is relatively small but reflects the fact that the population is only 22 per cent urbanized (CIA 2012, p. 673). The average woman has 6.7 children and the population growth is three per cent per year.

South Sudan in recent years has had the highest maternal mortality rate in the world with its rate being estimated at 2000 per 100,000 maternities'. The UN commented 'In South Sudan, a 15-year-old girl is more likely to die in childbirth than to complete her education' (IRIN 2012a). However, there have been some positive developments. The Government hopes that improved education and health will bring down child and maternal mortality rates. Contraception can also improve health. A UN affiliate commented:

> At Gurei clinic on the outskirts of the capital, Juba, women crowd into a makeshift shelter set up to give talks on birth spacing and limiting. Shushing babies and quieting older children, women who never knew there was a way to control births when they arrived are engrossed as health workers explain methods. (IRIN 2012a)

Some men oppose their wives using contraception because large families may be prized. There are sometimes angry exchanges between husbands and staff.

However, health workers reported that awareness was increasing and that men were coming round to the idea that small families also have a value (ERIN 2012a).

One widely quoted estimate from 2012 was that less than two per cent of women of child bearing age use modern contraception. With prevalence being so restricted there will be some who seek abortion. One such was 'Joyce' who was the only girl in her school to have completed primary education. She became pregnant and contracted HIV. She said 'A man offered me money to have sex. I did not know what contraception was … my parents allowed me to study instead of marriage so I was even more frightened to tell them'. She sought the help of a traditional healer who attempted to induce an abortion and left her bleeding. Her parents took her to the hospital where the abortion was completed, although it took two months for her to be released. At the age of 22 she now visits a family planning charity for her contraception.

Sudan

The population was estimated at 34.2 million in 2011 and its life expectancy at birth was 62.6 years. Its religion is 70 per cent Sunni Muslim 25 per cent indigenous beliefs and five per cent Christian (mainly in the south). In the year 2011 the birth rate was 31.7 per 1,000 and the death rate 8.3. The rate of natural increase of population was 1.9 per cent in 2011 the and average woman had 4.2 children. The capital city is Khartoum with a population of 5.0 million in 2009 (CIA 2012, p. 685).

In 1983 the Government tried to institute Islamic law throughout the country. This led to riots throughout the South and in the following year a state of emergency. Sudan supported Iraq's invasion of Kuwait in 1991 and in 1995 the UN endorsed an accusation that the country was sheltering the Islamic militants who had attempted to assassinate Egypt president Hosni Mubarak. In 1998 the US launched cruise missiles at Khartoum to retaliate for the bombing of its embassies in Tanzania and Kenya and to destroy what it said was a chemical weapons factory (Wright 2006, pp. 678–9). The country has also been torn apart by civil war in the South and West during which many women have been raped. This led to Fetters commenting 'Violence is systematically used as a weapon of war by the Janjaweed – a gross breach of international humanitarian law.' She continues to maintain that around one in twenty women suffering rape become pregnant but that this is not the only possible problem. Women may also be rejected by their husbands and have to suffer pelvic inflammatory disease or HIV infection. The law in the Sudan does allow abortion to save the life of the woman and for rape if it is requested by the woman not more than 90 days after the offence occurred. (Fetter 2006). Research published in 1999 stated that abortion was common in Western Dinka which is in south-west Sudan.

Contraceptive use has been low and, for example, in North Sudan only used by one in ten (9 per cent) of married women in the year 2,000 (UN 2004, p. 57)

Tanzania

The unification of territories led to the formation of the country in 1964. One-Party rule ended in 1995 with the restoration of democratic elections. Its population was 43.6 million in July 2012. Its religion is 35 per cent Muslim, 35 per cent indigenous beliefs and 30 per cent Christian. In the year 2011 the birth rate was 31.8 per 1,000 and the death rate 11.9 and rate of natural increase was 2.0 per cent. This rate of increase has reduced from 3.2 per cent during 1990–1995 (Population Division 2007). In 2011 the average woman had 4.0 children which is a reduction from 4.7 in 2005 (Wright 2006, p. 483). The capital city is Dar es Salaam with a population of 3.2 million in 2009 (CIA 2012, p. 717).

The economy took a downturn in the 1990s due to a number of factors including the debt problem, Rwandan refugees and general economic malaise. This led to a worsening of sexual and reproductive health facilities for women. We have seen that the country has had a relatively high maternal mortality rate. It is four times the maternal mortality rate of Latin America and almost fifty times as high as the rates of the industrial countries. In 2012 the mayor of New York, Michael Bloomberg conducted a press conference with the president of Tanzania Jakaya Kikwete. They announced an innovative project to reduce death in childbirth. One aspect of the initiative was to build clinics and train health personnel in isolated rural areas. They felt that this model of action could be helpful in other countries (Population Matters 2012).

In 1959 the Family Planning Association of Tanzania was set up in Dar es Salaam. It came to be known as UMATI and grew to have national coverage. It said that it was going to concentrate on providing help to parents. This approach aimed to negate some of the criticism that promoting contraception would encourage promiscuity amongst the young. The development of contraceptive services led to an increase in the percentage of women using modern methods from 10.4 per cent in 1991 to 25.4 per cent in 1999. In 2012 President Kitwete said that the rate of usage was just under a quarter (24 per cent). However, he hoped to increase it to three in five (60 per cent) at which level the population would be at replacement level. (Population Matters 2012).

A *Lancet* article presented research proposing that meeting contraceptive needs could cut maternal deaths by a third and that contraception was already cutting the number of maternal deaths by half (Tavernise 2012). Melinda Gates also suggested that contraception substantially reduced the number of unsafe abortions (Weinberger 2012).

In the 1990s the high rate of breastfeeding helped keep the pregnancy and abortion rate down and in 1991–92 the median length of breastfeeding was 21 months (Mturi and Hinde 2001). The abortion law in Tanzania follows the 1861 British law together with the liberalization of the 1938 Bourne judgment and subsequent developments which allow the protection of the physical or mental health of the woman (Francome 1984). As this law is relatively restrictive there are many unsafe abortions. In Tanzania in 1993, the cost per day of post-abortion care was over seven times the annual amount allowed by the Ministry of Health for per capita health expenses (Brookman-Amissah and Moyo 2004). A 1987 study in Dar es Salaam surveyed 300 women who were in hospital after early pregnancy loss. It found that 31 per cent had had an induced abortion (Population Divison 2007) An innovative study was concerned with the role of the male partners at the time of the abortion. In 2005 it reported that of 213 men accompanying their partners 44 per cent of single men and 81 per cent of married men had used birth control. In part this will have been due to age and the figures are relatively small but it does suggest a need to spread contraceptive information to the unmarried. This study also proposed that there was a need for men to be more involved in post abortion counselling in the hope that the contraception usage will be increased and the abortion rate reduced (Rasch and Lyaruu 2005).

Marie Stopes Tanzania (MST) provides a high proportion of the Family Planning activities in Tanzania and many of the sterilizations.

Togo

The population was estimated at 7.0 million in 2012. In 2011 Its life expectancy at birth was 63.2 years which is a nine years increase since the period 2000–2005 when it was 54 years. Its religion is 51 per cent indigenous beliefs 29 per cent Christian and 20 per cent Muslim. In the year 2011 the birth rate was 35.3 per 1,000, the death rate 7.8. The average woman had 4.6 children (CIA 2012, p. 728). The use of contraception was less than one in five (17 per cent) of the fertile population (15–49).

Induced abortion is still a criminal act in Togo, punishable under a law based on the French 1920 Act banning incitement to commit an abortion and anti-conception propaganda. In 1981, the government promulgated a new penal code which was based on the law of 1920, with a few minor modifications. In 2006 it legalized abortion in the case of rape or incest. The decision to terminate the pregnancy is taken by a panel of three doctors. This limited provision only concerns a very limited number of cases and so do not substantially reduced illegal abortion rates.

There is condemnation of abortion on the part of the religious authorities. The data that does exist is taken from hospital statistics and medical studies concerned with the complications of abortion or from studies of young people. The hospital statistics reveal that a large proportion of maternal mortality is the result of induced abortions. At the university hospital in Lomé, a study of 191 maternal deaths in 1991 showed that in 32 per cent of these deaths, the initial cause was an induced abortion. In 1996, a study carried out in the Central and Maritime regions with a sample of 1,854 schoolgirls (in their last five years at school), showed that 23 per cent had already been pregnant and that 86 per cent of these pregnancies were ended by an induced abortion and that eight per cent of cases ended with the removal of the uterus because of complications (Toussa-Ahossu 1991).

A 1996 study on the prevalence of pregnancies among students in Togo aged from 12 to 26 showed that 84 per cent of these schoolgirl pregnancies ended in an induced abortion. According to other studies involving female clients of family planning centres and pupils, 24 per cent of the female clients and 23 per cent of the pupils said that they had had at least one abortion (Amergee 1999). Finally, a study in 2001 involving 3,459 women, from all over Togo, observed that nine per cent said that they had had at least one abortion (19 per cent in Lomé). However, this figure seems low in comparison with other information. State hospitals as well as religious and private hospitals treat the complications produced by induced abortions. Curettage has been the method mainly used but MVA has begun to be used too (for example, at the university hospital in Lomé). The providers are gynaecologists and GPs, medical assistants and occasionally nurses. These groups also offer abortion in certain medical practices and private clinics but they remain illegal.

There is the joint activity of the government (Ministry of Social Action) and the civil society (Group for Reflection and Action, Women Democracy and Development and Women in Law and Development in Africa) for a general improvement in the legislation relating to sexual and reproductive health, and the development of a family code more favourable to the condition and rights of women.

Tunisia

The population was estimated at 10.7 million in 2011 and its life expectancy at birth was 75.2. Its religion is 98 per cent Muslim, one per cent Christian and one per cent Jewish and other religion (CIA 2012, p. 738). In the year 2011 the birth rate was 17.3 per 1,000 and the death rate 5.9. The rate of natural increase is 1.1 per cent. This is below half the rate of increase in 1985 which was 2.6 per cent. The Tunisian Government has achieved significant results, with the total fertility rate decreasing from 7.2 children per woman in 1965 to 3.4 in 1991, 2.6 in 2000 and 2.0 children in 2011. Its capital is Tunis with a population of 659,000 in 2009 (CIA 2012, p. 738).

Contraceptive use is high. It increased from half (53 per cent) of married and cohabiting women in 1990 to seven out of ten (70 per cent) in the year 2,000 (UN 2004, p. 57). In 1965 Tunisia became the first Muslim country to liberalize its abortion law. The Tunisian Penal Code of 1913 and the legislative decrees of 1920 and 1940, which amended the abortion provisions of the Code, had all prohibited abortions except to save the life of the pregnant woman. A law of 1 July 1965 amended the Code to allow abortions to be performed during the first three months of pregnancy, if a couple had at least five living children, and at any time during pregnancy if the continuance of pregnancy posed a danger to the health of the pregnant woman. However, this law was regarded by many as being far too restrictive and so a more liberal one was passed. Tunisia's current abortion law dates from 1973 and it authorizes abortions on request during the first three months of pregnancy. After this period an abortion may be performed when there is a risk to the physical or mental health of the mother or that the unborn child will suffer from a serious disease or infirmity and abortion The performance of abortion is subsidized by the Government in the same way as all other medical services and those entitled to receive free health care can obtain an abortion free of charge in public hospitals.

The liberalization of abortion was part of a national policy directed to reducing fertility as a means of improving economic development. In 1973, when the new abortion law was approved, the 'Office National de la Famille et de la Population' was created to direct the family planning programme. Subsequently in 1988 legislative action was complemented by other measures intended to raise the status of women and decrease fertility. The country began providing schooling for both sexes and supported the right of women to practice contraception. It also uses the media to encourage family planning which was fully integrated into the basic health care system and specialized (maternal health) wards were created to provide abortions and other services.

IPPF reports (March 2007) that most recent data show the average Tunisian acceptor of family planning to be aged 30 years, have 3.7 living children and been married nine years. Although high parity is no longer a requirement to obtain an abortion, the majority of women have four or more children when they seek one. The 1996 rate of 8.6 abortions per 1,000 women aged 15–44 is remarkably low for a developing country. Although official statistics omit legal abortions performed in the private sector. The true rate is estimated to be around 11 per 1,000 women 15–44 which is still very low reflecting the family planning programme. Despite the success of the national family planning programme, acceptors enter the programmes at a relatively advanced age, indicating that contraception and abortion are used mainly to prevent subsequent births once the desired number of children has been reached.

Uganda

The population was estimated to be 35.9 million in 2012. Its life expectancy at birth was 53.5 years in 2011. Its religion is 42 per cent Catholic 42 per cent Protestant, 12 per cent Muslim and four per cent other or none(CIA 2012, p. 754) In the year 2011 the birth rate was 47.4 per 1,000 and the death rate 11.5. This gives a rate of natural increase of 3.6 per cent. In 2011 the average woman had 6.6 children which was the second highest in the world. The capital city is Kampala with a population of 1.5 million in 2009.

In 1995 a survey showed that only one in seven (14.8 per cent) of women were using contraception. This increased to nearly one in four (23 per cent) in the year 2,000 and around half these were modern methods (UN 2004, p. 57). This will have increased especially with the concern with HIV/AIDS. In fact, in 2007 MSI reported that it was selling three million condoms a month in the country and that during the World Cup tournament it toured the country in a bus promoting condoms to fans at football matches (MSI 2007b).

Abortion is illegal except to save the life of the woman. However, unsafe abortion is common with one estimate placing the figure at 300,000 a year for women aged 15–49. This provides an overall abortion rate of 54 per 1,000. Abortion is seen as shameful within the society and consequently women try to hide the fact that they have had one. However, despite this a study of 40 *bodabodamen* (motorcycle taxis) found that almost half their partners had had an abortion. A 40-year-old man told how he came to make his girlfriend pregnant and to her having an abortion:

> I went to her place and asked her for sex. She refused claiming she was not in her safe period. I was burning with passion so I convinced her that I was going to time (my ejaculation). I failed to withdraw because I was enjoying myself. She cried that I had impregnated her. She then checked the calendar to note the date and time that I had impregnated her. And that is what happened exactly. (Jagwe-Wadda, Moore and Wong 2006)

It is estimated that 20 per cent of women with complication from unsafe abortions do not seek treatment (Grimes 2006) this may be one of the reasons that one third of maternal deaths are due to unsafe abortion (Religious Tolerance 2005) Overall, it is estimated that 85,000 women are taken to hospital each year with the after effects of unsafe abortion (Jagwe-Wadda, Moore and Wong 2006). The difficulties faced can be gauged by a study in Mulago Hospital, Kampala from 1983–87. This found that the main problems faced were sepsis, haemorrhage and genital tract trauma. In 1993 a study in Kampala found that one in five of the maternal deaths was due to abortion. However, some women have minimal problems – a young woman told how she visited the abortionist. 'She boiled the herbs and gave me a bottle to drink, and the pregnancy stopped. The pregnancy was still young and so the drug given was not so strong'. Others experiences are much worse and when a 40-year-old urban male was asked why women did not seek help when they had post abortion problems he stated:

> It is because of ignorance. When the foetus comes out they do not get to know what remains inside. The daughter of a friend of mine died under similar circumstances. She fell very sick after stopping a pregnancy and she never sought treatment. By the time her father realized it and decided to take her for treatment it was too late and she died. (Jagwe-Wadda, Moore and Wong 2006)

There are social changes occurring. We mentioned the increased provision of condoms and furthermore, in 1995 the Demographic and Health Survey found that 29 per cent of births to those aged 15–49 were unplanned. However, by 2000 the percentage had increased to 38 per cent leading researchers to suggest that the target fertility had declined. (Jagwe-Wadda, Moore and Wong 2006).

Zambia

The population was estimated at 14.3 million in 2012 and its life expectancy at birth was 52.6 in 2011. Its religion is 50–75 per cent Christian 24–49 per cent Muslim and Hindu and one per cent traditional beliefs. In the year 2011 the birth rate was 43.5 per 1,000 which is the fourth highest in the world. The death rate was 12.4 per 1,000. This gives a rate of natural increase of 3.1 per cent. In 2011 the average woman had 5.9 children. The capital city is Lusaka with a population of 1.4 million in 2009 (CIA 2012, p. 815).

Data indicates over one quarter (27 per cent) of women in Zambia wanted contraception but did not have it (World Bank 2013). Dr Olgy Chitoma commented that there is an increase in demand and usage for contraception, However, there is concern about side effects, opposition from some partners and religious objections (Chakwe 2013). Planned Parenthood of Zambia is popular amongst the village women and one commentator states 'The average woman has six children. It make is easy to understand why women in the valleys of Naluyanda celebrated the arrival of Justin Kapila, the contraceptive man' (de Sam Lazaro 2004).

Some Christian groups propose abstinence as an alternative to the use of condoms and modern family planning methods to prevent unwanted pregnancies and HIV. For example, Bishop Banda was quoted 'We can increase young people's ability to postpone sexual involvement until they are married (Religion and Ethics 2004). This abstinence approach is one put forward by the US right as part of a solution to the HIV/AIDS epidemic, The US funds for HIV/AIDS in Zambia increased six times under the Republicans but the overall aid for Family Planning has started small and has decreased. However, the country has received funds from the Japan International Co-operation Agency (Population Division 2007).

Abortion in Zambia is based on the 1972 Act which follows the wording of the British law and states 'Abortion is allowed when the continuance of the pregnancy would involve risk to the life of the pregnant woman greater than if the pregnancy were terminated'. In my earlier book *Abortion Freedom* (1984, p. 99) I pointed out that with this wording professionals realize that as childbirth is more dangerous than abortion, the latter is always legal in the early stages. However, observers state that the average person in Zambia does not realize that abortion could be available. There are also many obstacles to legal abortion. These include economic factors. According to one observer an illegal operation may only cost a dollar while a legal one may be around 12 dollars. There are also other obstacles such as the need to have three doctors to sign the form. A study of five important hospitals from 2003–2008 found there had been 616 legal abortions. The same hospitals found that over the period there were 52,791 women admitted for complications from abortion. So there were around 85 times as many women admitted outside the legal sector (Mushabati 2012).

Further information is provided by Rose Hoban who spent time in Zambia and published her findings in 2009. She reported:

> Abortion is legal in Zambia as long as it is provided in a medical setting by a medical practitioner. But the procedure is so stigmatized women don't talk about it. Many women do not know that it is legal or how or where to get an abortion done safely. (Admin 2009)

She quoted Iness Kabanda, a leading midwife in Lusaka, who said that many women who could not organize a legal abortion made use of what potential abortifacients they thought were available. These included drugs but also grounds glass and even acid from batteries. Another observer quoted a 15-year-old with the pseudonym Agnes who was pregnant by her boyfriend:

> She thought about her parents, they were strict and she thought about what people would think of her. She went to see a retired nurse in one of the compounds. The nurse said she could perform the abortion at a fee, which she agreed to. According to Agnes the abortion was carried out and it was painful. She said the abortion still haunts her because she believes she committed a sin. (Chakwe 2007)

Some women report conflicts with their religion which can lead to them wishing to keep their termination a secret. One woman told Rose Hoban:

> I'm a Catholic – staunch Catholic ... and in the Catholic Church it is not allowed. But I'm doing it ... I'm breaking so many rules and of course I know God doesn't want this, but I just have to do it. (Admin 2009)

A gynaecologist in Luksaka – Stephen Mupeta – stated that 30 per cent of the maternal deaths in Zambia were from abortion and that he wanted to change it. At his hospital they used MVA and the hospital charged women only one dollar for the procedure (Admin 2009). Another piece of research found that 69 per cent of women knew someone who had died from an unsafe illegal abortion (Grimes et al. 2006).

The overall evidence for Zambia indicates a need for legal and bureaucratic changes to make abortion more easily obtainable. In the meantime one positive development has been the expansion of the availability of misoprostol which is commonly found in pharmacies and will reduce the demand for unsafe abortions (Mushabati 2012).

Zimbabwe

The population was estimated at 12.6 million in 2012. In 2011 the life expectancy from birth was 51.8 years which is low but much better than the period 2000–2005 when its life expectancy was estimated at 37 years (CIA 2012, p. 819, Wright 2006, p. 48). Its religion is 50 per cent syncretic (part Christian, part traditional), 25 per cent Christian, The country had gained its independence in 1980 under the Robert Mugabe. In 2000 he introduced a land distribution campaign which led to an exodus of White farmers and to widespread shortages of basic commodities (CIA 2012, p. 818).

In the year 2011 the birth rate was 32.2 per 1,000 and the death rate 12.4. This gives a rate of natural increase of 2.0 per cent. Its capital city is Harare with a population of 1.6 million in 2009 (CIA 2012, p. 819).

When the country gained its independence in 1980 the average woman had an average of almost seven children. A fertility survey in 1984 showed the average number of children was 6.5 per woman. This reduced to 3.8 in 2006. So over a period of 22 years the number of children had reduced by an average of 2.7 per woman. In 2011 the average woman had 3.6 children. Two observers commented that the reason for this was contraception. In 1980 only 14 per cent of married women aged 15–49 were using contraception. This increased to 60 per cent in 2005/6. This meant that only South Africa has better family planning than Zimbabwe in sub-Saharan Africa. Forty per cent of the women were on the pill (Akim and Kembo 2011).

It might seem surprising that the upheaval within the society did not lead to more disruption in family planning services. Akim and Kembo suggest that this was in large part due to the fact that family planning services were built on a solid foundation which was able to withstand the crisis. Furthermore, there has been an improvement in the status of women with education and an increasing right to own property. However, other observers do not paint such a rosy picture of the control of fertility in Zimbabwe. Frederick Sai, for example, saw maternity services in the society as problematical with one in 42 women dying in childbirth (Sai 2011). He also gives an example of a woman who could not get access to contraception:

> Rose is a mother of four with a fifth on the way. At a time when she should be eagerly awaiting the birth of her child she is instead worried about how to prevent her next pregnancy. She would like to wait at least two years, but she does not have any choice because she does not have access to family planning. (Sai 2011)

Frederick Sai said that she is not one in a million but rather one in 215 million women worldwide who do not have access to contraception.

There is evidence of widespread illegal abortion. One article was entitled ‘Our ugly secret: abortion in Zimbabwe, illegal but thriving’ (Sokwanele 2012). Others concur and in 2005 UNICEF estimated that there were 70,000 illegal abortions a year and that many methods were reported including the consumption of detergents, strong tea, malaria tablets, knitting needles and sharpened reeds. An example of the aftermath of an unsafe operation is reported. Grace was a mature, single mother with two children unable to face the birth of a third who she would not be able to support as follows:

> She begs him not to let her see the foetus, he's considerate enough to cover it with a paper towel as it lies in a bloody puddle at the end of the examination table, before helping her to her feet. When he returns to the leather armchair in his consulting room, she notices that he doesn't wash his hands before lighting a cigarette blowing smoke in her direction as she leans over the desk to hand him the money. 'Be careful not to tell anyone about this' he says 'the jails are full of women like you' ...there was clotting and cramps that had her balled up in pain in a corner of the sofa for the next two days, but, mostly she cried because of the agony of an infection which festered where the doctors unsterilized equipment had torn at her private parts. (Sokwenele 2012)

Grace was fortunate that the infection cleared after she was given antibiotics and a D&C. The infection cleared and the doctor treating her was discreet and did not report her to the police.

There is legal abortion in Zimbabwe, but there are great problems. The cost of a safe legal abortion is around $350 (2012) which is beyond the means of the majority. The law on abortion is based on the Termination of Pregnancy Act 1977 which allows abortion on the grounds of the life of the woman, physical or mental defects of the foetus and for rape and incest. However, obtaining one is problematic. For example, Mildred Mapingure was raped in the course of a robbery in 2007 and the delays in her having a legal abortion were such that it was deemed too late for her to have a termination. Consequently she had to continue with the pregnancy (*Staff Reporter* 2012).

Summary

The evidence shows that Africa has particular problems with family planning as part of wider problems of the health of the continent. The tensions created may be one factor in the cause of wars. There is a great opportunity for governments on this continent to make important improvements to the lifestyle of its population and for the richer countries to help in this endeavour.

Chapter 5
Latin America and the Caribbean

> 'Police handcuffed Coutino still bleeding from the abortion to the hospital bed. Later in the day they booked her into Rio de Janiero's notorious Bangu prison'.

Abortion laws in Latin America and the Caribbean are among the most restrictive in the world with some countries not even allowing abortion to save the life of the woman. There are a few exceptions, for example, Puerto Rico which has strong links with the US and comes under its law. Cuba gives legal abortion on request within the first three months of pregnancy. Barbados, Colombia, Guyana and most recently Uruguay allow legal abortion under a variety, if somewhat limited range of circumstances. Nevertheless, estimates are that over nine out of ten abortions in the region are illegal. Even when abortion is legally permitted, for example for rape, safe abortion services are often inaccessible. This is especially true for women who are poor, young, or live in rural areas. It has led to the rate of unsafe abortions being higher in Latin America and the Caribbean than any other region of the world.

Facts on unsafe abortion

The estimated number of abortions in the region increased from 4.1 million to 4.4 million between 2003 and 2008. Overall in the region, 95 per cent of the abortions are unsafe. In the Caribbean it is below half (46 per cent) but in Central and South America virtually all abortions are unsafe (Guttmacher Institute 2013). Around one million women in Latin America and the Caribbean are hospitalized annually for treatment for the consequences of unsafe abortion. The most common problems are excessive blood loss, infection and incomplete abortions. There are some very serious complications that can occur such as perforation of internal organs, septic shock and inflammation of the peritoneum. Fortunately these are less common. Because poor and rural women have to depend on less safe methods and on untrained providers they are more likely to face severe complications. In fact experts in Guatemala and Mexico estimate that around a half of poor women having an abortion face complications needing medical treatment (Guttmacher Institute 2012).

Misoprostol is obtained from a variety of sources and has increased the safety of illegal abortions. It has been especially common in Brazil, Colombia, Dominican Republic, Ecuador, Mexico and Peru (Guttmacher Institute 2012). Other countries such as Haiti are showing increased usage as we shall see.

There has been a pattern in that Western countries colonized the region and introduced harsh laws making abortion illegal. They then left and changed their own laws so that native women could get good treatment. However, they left the women of the colonized countries facing severe restrictions. We shall see that

Haiti is a case in point. Abortion is still banned under a French law dating back to 1810 and women have problems accessing safe treatment. Yet the French, like other colonial powers have now liberalized their laws so that their women have the right to choose in the early months of pregnancy.

There has been a movement for change however, and the campaign for the widespread decriminalization of abortion in Latin America and the Caribbean began in 1990. As mentioned there have been a few successes in making changes but there has been a great amount of opposition especially from the Catholic Church. Some activists have suggested that the rest of the world has not been sufficiently aware of the difficulties women face. For example Gillian Kane, IPAS policy adviser commented in September 2012 'Few people realize that women actually go to jail' (Information from ICWRSA 27 September). However, there is evidence of some countries turning a 'blind eye' to abortion. As early as October 2003 a six month study of women's experiences of receiving medical abortion under clinical supervision was carried out in Mexico, Colombia, Ecuador and Peru. This found that 22 out of the 49 women in the study had never used a modern method of contraception. Consequently, it indicated that improvement in education in family planning was very much needed on the continent (Lafaurie 2005). Things have improved since then and the population increase has reduced. In the period 1970–1975 the average number of children was 5.0 per woman. It fell to 3.7 in the period 1995–2000 (UN 2004, p. 29). In large part this must have been due to illegal abortions and an estimate in 2010 suggested there were 4 million illegal abortions each year in Latin America (Gutierrez 2010). The country by country figures in Latin America and the Caribbean for maternal mortality and infant mortality rates are provided in Table 5.1. Overall, the main method of contraception on the continent has been female sterilization and in 1997 three in ten females were sterilized. One in seven (14 per cent) were using the pill. Although the region is predominantly Catholic only one in twenty were using the rhythm method (UN 2004, p. 47).

On the 22 May 2011, a hotline was started. Activists in Venezuela began to teach women about misoprostol and so followed a path trodden by Argentina, Chile, Peru and Ecuador. Women in Venezuela were told they could call a telephone number and receive information as to how to safely use the drug for abortion purposes. This movement suggests that it will be increasingly difficult for anti-abortion legislation to be enforced (Women on Waves 2011). There is also evidence that there has been a reduction in the harmful effects of illegal abortion as we shall see in the country by country analysis.

An important point about Latin American in particular is the strength of the Catholic Church. In Europe, religion failed to stop nominally Catholic countries such as Italy and France from decriminalizing abortion in the early months of pregnancy. However, in Latin America it has used all its power to restrict abortion rights. One observer commented that the region had felt a 'fundamentalist offensive by the Catholic Church to keep Latin America a land free of abortions – legal ones at least' (Gutierrez 2010).

Table 5.1 The 29 countries of Latin America and the Caribbean (2011)

	Maternal mortality rate per 100,00	Infant mortality rates per 1,000	Population millions
	2010	2013	2013 (July, est.)
Central America			
Belize	53	20.8	0.3
Costa Rica	40	9.0	5.0
El Salvador	81	19.1	6.1
Guatemala	120	24.3	14.4
Honduras	100	19.3	8.4
Mexico	50	16.3	116.2
Nicaragua	95	21.1	5.8
Panama	92	11.0	2.4
South America			
Argentina	77	10.2	42.6
Bolivia	180	39.8	10.5
Brazil	56	19.8	201.0
Chile	25	7.2	17.2
Colombia	92	15.5	45.7
Ecuador	110	18.5	15.4
Guyana	280	33.5	0.7
Paraguay	99	21.5	6.6
Peru	67	20.9	29.8
Uruguay	29	9.2	3.3
Venezuela	92	19.8	28.5
Caribbean			
Bahamas	47	12.9	0.3
Barbados	51	11.1	0.3
Cuba	73	4.8	11.1
Dominican Republic	150	20.4	10.2
Haiti	350	50.9	9.9
Jamaica	110	14.0	2.9
Puerto Rico	20	8.0	3.7
St Lucia	35	12.1	0.2
Trinidad and Tobago	46	25.7	1.2
Virgin Islands	–	6.9	0.1

Note: The infant mortality rates measure deaths up to one year.
Source: CIA 2013, various pages (between p. 29 for Argentina and p. 795 for the Virgin Islands).

The UN subdivides the countries of Latin America into three regions. The list is largely of countries with populations above 300,000 and so does not include several smaller ones. It is instructive to consider the latest statistical data as to maternal and infant mortality rates. These are displayed in Table 5.1

Table 5.1 shows that Haiti has the highest maternal mortality rate with an estimated 350 deaths per 100,000 births, which is over four times the rate of the median of 77 for Argentina, and over 17 times the estimated death rate of 20 in Puerto Rico which has the lowest rate in the region (CIA 1913, p. 316). We shall see that countries with more liberal abortion laws tend to be the ones with the lowest maternal deaths. This is not surprising for we shall see that one Brazilian study found that almost half maternal deaths were due to unsafe abortions.

The data also shows a wide variation in infant mortality. Again the highest rate is Haiti with 50.9 deaths per 1,000 live births. Other countries with high rates are Bolivia (39. 8) and Guyana (33.5). The median rate is El Salvador with a rate of 19.1 which is under half the rate for Haiti. The lowest infant mortality rate is in Cuba (4.8) which has less than a tenth of the rate for Haiti. Other countries in the region with less than ten deaths per 1,000 births are the Virgin Islands (6.9), Chile (7.2), Puerto Rico (8.0), Costa Rica (9.0) and Uruguay (9.2).

The number of births per woman is higher than Europe but much less than Africa. No country in the region has a birthrate above four per woman and only five of the countries has an average of over three births per woman. These relatively low figures indicate that the local people do not follow the Catholic Churches' teaching on contraception and abortion. Let us consider the situation in the major countries of the region.

Argentina

Table 5.1 shows the population was estimated at 42.6 million in 2013 and its life expectancy at birth was 77.3 years. Its religion is nominally 92 per cent Catholic but less than 20 per cent are practising (CIA 2013, p. 29). Protestants and Jews both comprise two per cent of the population. The other four per cent are in other religions. In the year 2013 the birth rate was 17.1 per 1,000 and the death rate 7.4 per 1,000. This gives a rate of natural increase of 1.0 per cent. Its capital is Buenos Aires which had a population of 13.0 million in 2009. It was estimated that the average woman had 2.3 children in 2013 (CIA 2013, p. 29).

According to a law passed in the 1880s, strictly speaking abortion was illegal in all cases. However, exceptions were introduced in 1922 and penalties were suspended in two cases. The law was relaxed where the woman's life or health (including mental health) was threatened and also in the case of rape. The military removed these but when democracy was restored in 1984 they were reinstated except that now abortion for rape became legal only in the case of a mentally incapacitated woman. Presumably mentally competent women who become pregnant because of rape are meant to continue the pregnancy. A part of the country's hierarchy is close to the Vatican and in 1998 the President declared that 25 March was to be the 'day of the unborn child'. This is the day when Catholics celebrate the Annunciation – when Mary was supposedly told she would be the mother of the son of God. There are a number of vibrant women's groups in favour of abortion rights and modern contraception. These include the Catholic Women for the Right to Choose and the Women's Information Network of Argentina. In 2005 the twentieth Annual Meeting of Women's Organizations led to 30,000 marching for the right to choose. The health minister G. Garcia said he supported legalized abortion as did Carmen Argibay, who became the first woman appointed to the Argentinian Supreme Court (Mundoandino, accessed January 2014).

The law in Argentina is not adhered to and in 2007 the health minister estimated that there were 500,000 terminations a year, which would mean two in five pregnancies end in abortion. One woman told how she was offered an abortion for 250 pesos but she was told that the cost would be 300 if she wanted antibiotics. A second woman, 36 years old, first became pregnant at the age of 17 and had 10 children. She commented 'You seek all the ways out – pills anything. But if there is no way out then you take a knife or a knitting needle'. A third woman went with her friend who had an unwanted pregnancy: 'She went to the illegal clinic and she never came back. They said that it was a problem with the anaesthesia and she died in that very place. They said she died of a heart attack ... legally it was like nothing had happened' (Mundoandino, accessed January 2014). Observers report that women have tried to abort themselves with a variety of things 'rubber tubes, parsley sticks, knitting needles, and wood'. Many of these abortions are incomplete. Not surprisingly in recent years around 80,000 women have been hospitalized annually, which is about one in seven of all the abortions. Of course some women will be hesitant to have treatment for fear of being reported to the police. Those who do go to hospital may face difficult treatment and a social worker told Human Rights Watch (2007):

> A woman went to hospital with an abortion and she was infected and haemorrhaging. A doctor started to examine her and realized. He threw his instruments on the floor. He said "This is an abortion, you go ahead and die".

Things may have improved after research showed the poor quality of treatment and the lack of regard for women (Steel and Chiarotti 2004). There are signs that the Government may at last be recognizing the problem. It now provides free contraception for the poor although there are difficulties in accessing it.

Pressure to change the law has been exerted and on 28 May 2007 a group of 250 NGOs joined together to present a draft Bill calling for abortion on request up to 12 weeks with later exceptions for 'rape', 'grave foetal malformation' and problems with the 'physical or mental health' of the woman. Observers noted 'to date, no formal legislative debate has been conducted.' A change seemed nearer when in 2011 La Pampa province passed an abortion protocol which included access to contraception and abortion. This was, however, vetoed by the Governor despite the fact that in 2011 an opinion poll found that 45 per cent of people wanted women to be given the choice of an abortion up to 12 weeks. Four out of five supported abortion for rape (Mundoandino, accessed 17 January 2014).

In March 2012 there was a major liberalization when the Supreme Court decided that abortion should be allowed in the case of rape. Furthermore it decided that women would no longer have to seek judicial permission to get an abortion if they had been raped. A sworn statement to her doctor would be sufficient evidence (BBC News 2012).

In another case a 32-year-old woman who had been a sex slave until she escaped to a refuge, was refused an abortion. Her lawyer commented that her details were released to opponents of abortion. 'They shouted that she's a murderer and threatened her that if she continued that something really bad would happen to her'. The Supreme Court upheld her right to have an abortion and this case was used by some to argue for an extension in the law. Estal Diaz, for example, called for Argentina to give women the 'right to choose' (Warren 2012).

Barbados

The population was estimated at 288,725 in July 2013 and its life expectancy at birth was 74.8 years and has increased from 69 in 1970. Its religion is 71 per cent Protestant, four per cent Catholic and 21 per cent none or unspecified. Its capital city is Bridgetown with a population of 112,000 in 2009 (CIA 2013, p. 63). The Barbados abortion law used to follow the UK's Offences Against the Person Act (1861) with the change due to the 1938 Bourne Case which liberalized abortion for rape. In 1983 Barbados passed the Medical Termination of Pregnancy Act. This liberalized its law similar to the British 1967 Act. Under its terms abortion was allowed for a wide range of conditions including taking account of the pregnant woman's social and economic environment. Under the law, a pregnancy in the first 12 weeks could obtain approval for termination by one doctor. For pregnancies 12–20 weeks two doctors were needed and for those over 20 weeks three doctors were required. For these later pregnancies abortion would only be approved in the case of risk to the woman's life or 'grave permanent injury to the physical or mental health of the woman or her unborn child'.

So, although Barbados does not give women the expressed right to choose, its generally liberal position does mean that women generally have far more legal rights than exists in the vast majority of countries in the region. Consequently it does not have the health problems associated with unsafe abortion. Abortion still has public support (Francome and Vekemans 2007, p. 98).

Bolivia

The population was estimated at 10.5 million in 2013 and its life expectancy at birth was 68.2 years. Its religion is 95 per cent Catholic and (unusually) five per cent evangelical Methodist (CIA 2013, p.87). In the year 2013 the birth rate was 23.8 per 1,000 population and the death rate 6.7. The rate of natural increase is 1.7 per cent. Its capital La Paz had a population of 1.6 million (2009 estimate) (CIA 2013, p. 87).

The law on abortion was liberalized in 1973 to allow abortion for rape, incest and the curious case of 'abduction not followed by marriage' (Cohen 2012). Such a restrictive law meant that women had to go outside the legal system if they wanted a termination.

In addition to abortions on such grounds there is an illegal network. This was first systematically studied by researchers in 1983–84 who analysed the results of over 4,000 women who had experienced a problematic pregnancy loss. In the sample 23 per cent had a legal abortion and 77 per cent an illegal one. The death rate was six per 1,000 women who had had an abortion and only 0.3 per 1,000 amongst those having a miscarriage. Only seven per cent of the women had used a modern method of contraception in the month before they became pregnant. This led to the authors suggesting that there was great need to improve family planning services (Bailey et al. 1988).

In 2007 Friedman-Rudovsky discussed the fact that many left wing groups were not pushing for abortion rights. He proposed this was in large part because of concern with the Catholic Church. However, he also drew attention to the fact that such things as gay rights or abortion rights were seen as part of the 'imperialist agenda of the industrialized world.' He maintained that the country had 80,000 abortions a year. If correct this would be a very high number for a country with a population of under nine million. He also estimated four hundred of these women would die of illegal abortion each year. His information was that the prices at the time were $150 for a safe abortion and $50 for a 'back alley' one (Friedman-Rudovsky 2007). The figure of 400 annual deaths may well be an overestimate as the WHO estimated a much lower number.

In 2012 observations on the provision of illegal abortion were published. One example was a centre which called itself a 'Dentista'. However, the observer, Naomi Cohen, commented that the generally poor condition of the premises suggested that the man in the white coat would not be holding a toothbrush. She continued:

> Bolivia may produce fifty thousand tons of coffee leaves each year but the clandestine and most dangerous marker is behind these closed doors. The patient is one of an estimated 100–250 women a day in Bolivia who receive an abortion (Cohen 2012)

She continued to say that there is a witches market where a woman can purchase the ingredients for an abortifacient (fig leaves, oregano, and seaweed). Overall abortion was the causes of one third of the maternal deaths and the evidence suggested that one half of Bolivian women had had to deal with unwanted pregnancies. The local organization Bolivian Catholics for the Right to Decide is active in trying to change the law (Cohen 2012).

Brazil

The population was estimated at 201.0 million in 2013 and its life expectancy at birth was 73.0 years. Its religion is 74 per cent per cent Catholic but many people are inactive. In the year 2013 the birth rate was 15.0 per 1,000 and the death rate 6.5 per 1,000. This gives a rate of natural increase of 0.9 per cent The 2009 estimates found its capital Brazilia had a population of 3.8 million which was much smaller than either Sao Paulo 20.0 million or Rio De Janeiro 11.8 million (CIA 2013, p. 100) Contraceptive use in Brazil is high with four out of five (80 per cent) of women of childbearing age using it. The average woman has 1.8 children (2013 est.) (CIA 2013, p. 100).

Fred De Sam Lazaro (2011) commented that 'Brazil's plummeting birthrate would seem like a triumph for the countries women's movement'. He continued to comment that the world's largest Catholic country nevertheless had a situation where 80 per cent of women of childbearing age used contraception. This resulted in the birth rate falling from six children per woman in 1960 to 1.9 in 2011 (1.8 in 2013). The Government has been supportive of contraception and for many years has been giving condoms out at carnival time. This approach brought it at odds with the Vatican. In 2007 the Pope visited Brazil and called upon Catholics to maintain traditional family values and also made it clear that the Vatican believed that the Government's official health programmes were encouraging promiscuity. Two weeks after the visit President da Silva announced a plan to heavily subsidize the birth control pill so that it would be available in 3,500 private drug stores at only 20 cents a month. He stated the 'programme would give the poor the same rights as the wealthy to have the number of children they want' (Duffy 2007). In addition the health minister Jose Temporao commented 'If men got pregnant the issue would be resolved' (Perraza 2008).

As far as abortion is concerned the law is based on the 1940 Penal Code and allows it to save the life of the woman or for rape. However, even women who have been raped do not find it easy to obtain a legal abortion. One observer commented 'although sexual violence is highly prevalent, legal abortion in cases of rape is rarely performed in public hospitals. This means that a large number of women who should have access to safe abortion in a hospital environment are risking their lives by being forced to resort to clandestine abortions' (Faundes et al. 2004). In fact during the period 1978–1987 at one Brazilian hospital abortion complications accounted for 47 per cent of maternal deaths (Population Information Program 2007, p. 1) There was no official sanction of abortion for foetal abnormality so when in July 2004 a judge decided to allow an abortion for anencephaly, a storm broke leading to the Catholic Church strongly challenging the ruling and the case going to the Supreme Court, There the judges voted 7–4 to set aside the ruling. So the law is very restrictive and in 2004 the country only had 140 legal abortions registered (Ross 2005).

Although legal abortions are few there are many unsafe abortions. It was in August 1986 that Cytotec (misoprostol) was approved for sale over the counter.

The word of its abortifacient properties spread until in July 1991 the Brazilian ministry of health imposed restrictions (Arilha and Barbosa 1993). This meant that many women seeking abortions had to return to the traditional methods. Also in 1991 the Guttmacher Institute estimated that the country had 1.4 million abortions (with a range of from 1.0 million to 2.0 million). This number would result in an abortion rate of 41 per 1,000 women 15–44 and one quarter of pregnancies ending in abortion (Henshaw et al. 1999). Dulce Xavier of Brazil's chapter of Catholics for a Free Choice commented:

> Here in Brazil, women sometimes ingest a poison used to kill rats ... It's a dramatic situation and the women who die as a result of clandestine abortions in Brazil are mainly young, black and poor. Women with money can pay to have an abortion in a private clinic. (Ross 2005)

Over 4,000 Brazilian gynaecologists were asked about their personal experience of abortion. Almost a quarter of female and a third of male obstetricians had faced an unwanted pregnancy and four out of five of these were aborted (Faundes et al. 2004, p. 47). Even amongst those to whom religion was 'very important', still 70 per cent of unwanted pregnancies were aborted. Observers have reported the individual problems women have faced. Ross highlighted a woman only identified as Martha, a 26-year-old mother, who had been raped by her estranged husband. Marital rape not being recognized in Brazilian law, her husband threatened to report her to the police. Nevertheless, she could not face continuing the pregnancy under these circumstances. She used misoprostol which precipitated the abortion but left her bleeding for forty days. She did not go to the hospital for fear of being prosecuted. Another woman had greater problems. In the fall of 2002, Viviane Coutino, a breastfeeding mother, became pregnant again and also took misoprostol she became ill and checked into hospital where the following occurred:

> An attending physician was angry about the steady stream of abortions he was seeing. He accused her of infanticide a crime carrying a possible six year prison term. Police handcuffed Coutino still bleeding from the abortion to the hospital bed. Later in the day they booked her into Rio de Janeiro's notorious Bangu prison. She spent nearly two months in jail. She never knew who was caring for her 10-month-old son. She said 'I could not believe this was happening. I thought only about my son'. (Hall 2003)

Although, poor women may fall foul of the law, in Brazil there is a network of doctors providing abortions for richer women. When considering the role of abortifacients drugs observers noted that there were separate gynaecologists for general needs and for abortions. In part this was because doctors performing abortions have to 'pay police in order to obtain a corrupt form of authorization' (Arilha and Barbosa 1993, p. 45).

There has been some liberalization in the practice of the law. At one time the woman had to file a complaint to the police in order to obtain an abortion for rape. This requirement has now been removed. In 2005 the Government appointed an 18-member commission which recommended that abortion should be made legal in the first three months of pregnancy. This raised a great amount of opposition (Perazza 2008). In 2010 Downie quoted a study that one in five women of child bearing age had obtained an abortion and commented that abortion was almost routine in Brazil quoting Macella Medeiros:

> The woman who has an abortion is a Brazilian woman. She could be your cousin, your mother, your sister or your neighbour, all the evidence shows that this is a serious problem and one which is not being debated openly.

It is not surprising that the government has come into conflict with the Catholic Church on a number of occasions. One such occurred in 2008 when the government mindful of the risks of the spread of HIV/AIDS and unwanted pregnancy decided to give away nearly 20 million condoms during carnival. The Government also decided to provide post-coital contraception (Perazza 2008) In 2009 a nine-year-old girl was raped by her stepfather and became pregnant. She obtained a legal abortion, however, her mother was then excommunicated by the Catholic Church (De Sam Lazaro 2011) In 2010 the Pope approved the use of condoms amongst gay men to stop the spread of HIV this may well be broadened to include heterosexuals using condoms within marriage to prevent disease (Thompson 2010).

In 2010 Downie stated that each year around 200,000 women are hospitalized because of the after-effects of abortion. Moraes (2011), stated that the high number of unsafe abortions has reduced the country's chance of meeting a UN Millennium Goal. The UN had set a target of countries reducing their maternal death rate by two thirds between 1990 and 2015. In Brazil the rate had halved by 2005 to 110 deaths per 100,000 births. Moraes suggested that since that time progress has been blighted by the high number of deaths from unsafe abortions (Moraes 2011). However, in the event Moraes fears were not realized. The target rate of 67 by 2015 was surpassed and the rate was down to 56 by 2010. This is likely to be because of the high rate of contraceptive usage and that misoprostol has made illegal abortions safer.

Generally in Brazil the police tolerate abortion despite it being illegal. However, a police raid on an abortion clinic was reported late on a Saturday night in January 2013. Eleven people were arrested (Rapoza 2013). So the situation is still in flux.

Caribbean Islands of Anguilla, Antigua, St Kitts, St Martin and Sint Maarten

These five countries are relatively small with a total population of about 200,000 and they are situated in the Northeast Caribbean. St Martin and Sint Maarten

(French) is a two country Island where the researchers began working and as the project developed, the other countries were added. Anguilla is a British Overseas Territory while Antigua is part of a two-island country of Antigua and Barbuda which has been independent since 1981. St Kitts is one of the two islands in St Kitts and Nevis independent since 1983 (Pheterson and Azize 2005). Research was thorough. They carried out in depth interviews with 25 doctors; 16 carried out abortions, only two of them complying with legal guidelines. They also interviewed health professionals, advisors or government officials including a Minister of Health and an Attorney General (Pheterson and Azize 2005, p. 45).

At Sint Maartin the researchers went to the Woman's Desk which is a government community Centre and were told:

> Abortion is illegal in Sint Marten … no the law is not a problem … . Everyone knows who is doing them. We don't talk about it, we can't talk about it since it is illegal and we are a Government agency. Abortion is a taboo here. (Pheterson and Azize 2005, p. 46)

A physician told them that abortion was tolerated because people realized it was legal in Holland. Another respondent, who provided aspiration abortions, told how an inspector from the ministry of health inspected and all they did was asked about his technique. He commented 'They know it is a needed service'. A fourth doctor commented that he was not in favour of legalization because it would lead to greater bureaucracy and delays. 'The system works fine the way it is'. In the French part of the Island the service depended on French law and was the only one of the five countries to provide Medical abortion with the combination of mifepristone and misoprostol. However, at the time of the study these had to be carried out in a hospital rather than at home or in a doctor's office. In 2004 French practice changed to allow doctors to supervise medical abortions until 49 days since last menstrual period. The researchers did report that some migrant women were buying misoprostol from underground distributors who carried the drug from one island to another. Also some local residents told that women from Anguilla would go to St. Martin to avoid trouble from their church which might expel them if it were discovered. Anguilla had in fact recently changed its law before the research began but it does not seem that the liberalization had much effect on practice at the time.

In Antigua abortion remained illegal, although it was carried out openly. A nurse who had learned to do manual vacuum aspiration said that once abortions were carried out by unskilled operators:

> People used to end up with sepsis really sick, and when I say sick I have seen times you had to stay outside the room the smell was so bad. You don't see that anymore. Doctors realised that people were dying or becoming infertile and they decided was inhumane to let people suffer like that … now people go to the doctors and the doctors help them. The Church, doesn't say anything about it

> because it isn't legal … but its done as a cloak and dagger thing, its done more or less openly and safely. (Pheterson and Azize 2005)

One gynaecologist described how when doctors went to the Government to try and change the law they said 'Look, it hasn't been a problem, what we do is turn a blind eye, but to legislate would cause too much a problem with the Church'. Another respondent, who was a health administrator for a non-governmental organization, said he thought the country was not ready for reform and expressed the view that stirring up a debate by damage the provision of services (Pheterson and Azize 2005, p. 48).

Another gynaecologist told how he had worked in many of the English speaking Caribbean Islands and abortion was not legal in most of them with Barbados and Guyana being exceptions. However, he commented 'It's tolerated because nobody is going to prosecute a doctor' (Pheterson and Azize 2005, 48). In May 2005 the researchers organized a conference in Antigua–Barbuda on 'Safe abortion in the Caribbean: From Law to Practice'. Participants attended from 14 Caribbean countries including Barbados, Curacao, Dominica, Guadeloupe, Guyana, Jamaica, St Eustatius, Puerto Rico, St Kitts-Nevis, St Lucia and Trinidad–Tobago. The Conference called for a decriminalization of abortion in the Caribbean.

Chile

In 2013, life expectancy at birth was 78.3 years and the number of children per woman was below replacement rate at 1.8 (CIA, 2013, p. 149). In the 2002 census its religion was 70 per cent Catholic and nearly one in five (17.2 per cent) Protestant. In the year 2013 the birth rate was 14.1 per 1,000 and the death rate 5.9 per 1,000. This gives a rate of natural increase of 0.8 per cent (CIA 2013, p. 149).

Chile is one of the countries which does not officially allow abortion to save the life of the woman. It was based on the 1874 penal code which would not allow abortion for any reason. In 1931 there was liberalization and abortion was allowed to save the woman's life. However, in 1989 General Pinochet's regime annulled even this minor liberalization. During the presidential elections of 1999 President Lagos supported abortion to save the life of the woman and for her health. However, he later retracted this position (Human Rights Watch 2007a). We saw in the introduction that at least until 1935 the Catholic Church did not allow abortion for an ectopic pregnancy. It subsequently changed its view. However, it does not seem that the Chilean Government has acted on it. For observers state that the law will not allow an immediate abortion 'the law requires waiting until the final stages of pregnancy before termination'.

One such case was that of Claudia Pizarrio a woman suffering from cancer. She was carrying an anencephalic baby and was forced to continue the pregnancy. Her baby lived for one hour, fifteen minutes. A second woman Karen Espindola was faced with carrying a potential baby whose brain was not properly formed.

She wanted a termination but was forced to continue a very unhappy pregnancy (Bonnefoy 2009).

There have been reductions in the maternal mortality rates and in the period 1990–2000 the rate fell by 60.3 per cent and a large but unspecified part of this drop will have been due to a reduction in deaths from unsafe abortion. However, although deaths from unsafe abortion have reduced, they are still much higher than elsewhere and women are facing great difficulties. Ross reports the case of 16- year-old Monica Maureira admitted to hospital haemorrhaging who commented 'I remember the nurses telling me that if I did not give them the name of the doctor who gave me the abortion, then they would let me bleed to death (Ross 2006).

It appears there is still a great problem with teenage pregnancy and Ross reported that many girls were pregnant at a very young age. This fact seems to have led on 30 January 2006 to the president Michelle Bachelet legalizing the 'morning after' pill for teenagers without parental consent. However, this law was set aside later in the year at the Santiago Court of Appeals when opponents argued that there should be parental consent for the ages 14–18 years (Ross 2006) The court then changed its mind and it seems the pills are once more allowed without consent. It could help reduce the number of unsafe abortions.

An important ten-year project led by Ramiro Molina of the University of Chile introduced contraception, counselling, and education to three poor communities. This led to an 82 per cent drop in the abortion rate in some areas. This project has been used as an example of what could be done to improve women's health (Ross 2006). Although Chile is strongly Catholic a study found that over four out of five (81.3 per cent) Catholics were in favour of artificial contraception (CIA 2007). So a push for modern contraceptive coverage may find support. There is less possibility of abortion liberalization. Estrada (2006) wrote an article entitled 'Chile: therapeutic abortion a distant but not impossible prospect.' In this she pointed out that activists fighting for liberalization faced a difficult situation with zero political support, the opposition of the Catholic Church and limited public support. However, she noted the importance of the 1979 UN General Assembly 'Convention on the elimination of all forms of discrimination against women' (CEDAW). Chile ratified this in 1989.

A great deal of controversy was caused in 2012 when an article by Dr Elard Koch was published. He and his colleagues argued that the tightening of the law led to a reduction in the number of abortions and did not lead to an increase in the maternal mortality rates because of an increase in clandestine abortions. He argued that there was over a ninety per cent reduction in abortion induced maternal deaths since prohibition in 1989 (Kotch 2012).

Joyce Arthur, in criticizing the work of Koch, pointed out that women in hospital were hardly likely to admit that they had committed the offence of having an abortion. Joyce Choice, pointed out that Koch was a member of a conservative group called 'We care' and said his research was a disgraceful example of BAD science (Biased, Agenda Driven).

In 2009 there was an important development with the formation of the Chilean safe abortion hotline which aimed to help women with illegal but safe misoprostol abortions This opened for four hours every day of the year and was run by volunteers some of whom had experienced adverse reactions following illegal abortions. One volunteer saw her roommate hospitalized and jailed for two years for carrying out an abortion with a television antenna. A review of its development said that the hotline was open seven days a week from 7–11 pm with 30 volunteers and by the beginning of 2013 had taken over 12,000 calls. Four other South American countries also had hotlines. These were Argentina, Ecuador, Peru and Venezuela (Nelsen 2013).

In 2012 Emily Anne forwarded an email which gave the phone number of the organization and provided details of a typical consultation:

> The woman on the other end explains that she has six pills of misoprostol and wants to know how to use them to induce an abortion … (and) I explain the symptoms and how to recognize problematic bleeding or infection.

She continued to say that lawyer's advice limited what she could say to callers without both of them risking three years imprisonment. However, the woman also wanted to know if a doctor would be at hand if she needed help. She was able to reassure the women that if the pill was taken from under the tongue then her symptoms would be identical to those of a miscarriage (Emily Anne, email 18 October 2012). This development and the spread of misoprostol will mitigate the effects of unsafe operations.

The International Campaign reported in September 2013 that the organization 'Feministra por el Aborto Seguro' and the School of Public Health from the local university convened a meeting to help promote safe abortion and decriminalization in Chile. It included Dr Anibal Faundes of Brazil and Dr Cristina Grela of Uruquay as well as activists from Chile.

There was a great amount of media coverage of a case where an 11-year-old girl had been repeatedly raped by her mother's boyfriend and was fourteen weeks pregnant. Amnesty International urged Chile to allow her to have an abortion. However, other reports stated that having abortion was not an option (*Telegraph* 2013) The report continued:

> The Roman Catholic Church retains a strong influence over society, although it has lost credibility since 2010 when four men alleged that they were abused by one of Chile's most revered priests when they were 14–17 years old. (*Telegraph* 2013)

The Catholic Church continues to risk losing credibility over sexuality. It is liberalizing but there is still a long way to go for it to have a practice of sexuality which is supportive of a good quality of life.

Colombia

The population was estimated at 45.7 million in 2013 and its life expectancy at birth was 75.0 years. Its religion is 90 per cent Catholic. In the year 2013 the birth rate was 17.0 per 1,000 and the death rate 5.3 per 1,000. This gives a rate of natural increase of 1.2 per cent. The average woman has 2.1 children (2013). Its capital Bogota has a population 8.7 million (2011, estimate) (CIA 2013, p. 161).

Contraceptive use increased from two thirds (66 per cent) married and cohabiting women in 1990 to 77 per cent per cent in the year 2,000 and of these 64 per cent were modern methods of contraception (UN 2004, p. 57).

The law of abortion in Colombia dates back at least to 1936 although the penalty was lower for women who had abortions 'to protect their honour' (Human Rights Watch 2007b). In 1979 Congresswoman Consuela Lleras unsuccessfully submitted a bill to legalize abortions on four grounds. These were for maternal health, rape, incest or foetal abnormality (Vieira 2005). Since then there have been several other bills, however, until Colombia was recognized as one of the countries in Latin America not to allow any abortions. This led to high numbers of illegal abortion and between 1985–89 unsafe abortion accounted for nearly one third of maternal deaths at one Colombian hospital.

However, despite the general illegality of abortion often being mentioned in the literature of those on both sides of the debate, the overall prohibition was softened in 1991 when four Constitutional Court judges commented about women pregnant through rape 'the exceptional and admirable thing would be for the woman to decide to continue the pregnancy until she gave birth … but she cannot be required to procreate, nor can she be the object of penal sanctions for having exercised her fundamental rights' (Francome and Vekemans 2007, p. 104).

In 2005 Monica Roa, a lawyer, with the support of the Spanish-based group 'Woman's Link Worldwide' challenged the law. On 10 May 2006, the Constitutional Court voted by 5–3 that abortion was not a crime under four conditions –maternal health, rape, incest or foetal abnormality. The bureaucratic conditions meant that it might still be difficult to obtain a legal abortion. To obtain an abortion for rape the woman had to file a police report, and to obtain one on the grounds of health, she needed a medical certificate. The ruling explicitly stated that international laws take precedence over national ones. The Catholic Church excommunicated the five judges who voted for the change in the law (Caeser 2006). One of the cases that was given great publicity while the Court was considering its decision was that of Marta Gonzalez a 34-year-old mother of four children. Three weeks into her pregnancy she was diagnosed with cancer and wished to have an abortion so that she could have chemotherapy and radiation. However, this was refused by the authorities and as her pregnancy was logged in the system no private hospital would go against the decision. She had to face a lack of treatment (Caeser 2006).

The first abortion carried out under the act gained great publicity. An 11-year-old girl became pregnant after being raped by her stepfather. There were hundreds of opponents to the Act outside the hospital and the Catholic Church announced it was to excommunicate all those involved in the girls abortion including judges, physicians, nurses and the girl's parents. Senator Gina Parody commented 'The Vatican has the right to excommunicate whoever it likes. But I hope that it also excommunicates priests when they rape boys or girls (Brodzinsky 2006).

In 1989 it was estimated that there were 289,000 abortions (with a range 288,000–404,000). In 2012 the figure of 400,000 was often mentioned. One calculation was that around 2006 a total of 36 per cent of teenager pregnancies ended in abortion compared to 12 per cent of pregnancies in married women (Human Rights Watch 2007c).

The women's movement had a success in September 2012 when the Colombian Constitutional Court ruled that Procurator Ordonez and two of his colleagues were not fulfilling their obligations to provide accurate data on reproductive rights (ICARSA document). Also there was a debate over the level of abortions when the conservative Chilean Do Koch criticized an estimate from the Guttmacher Institute in New York that Colombia had 400,000 abortions in 2008. He argued that it was nearer 22,000 (New 2012). This debate mirrors the one that had occurred in the UK much earlier (Francome 1976).

Costa Rica

Life expectancy at birth was 78.1 years (2013). Its religion is 76 per cent per cent Catholic and 16 per cent Protestant. In the year 2013 the birth rate was 16.3 per 1,000 and the death rate 4.4 per 1,000. This gives a rate of natural increase of 1.2 per cent. The average woman had 1.9 children San Jose, the capital, has a population of 1.5 million (2011 estimate) (CIA 2013, p. 175).

Abortion is allowed under a 1970 Act to protect the health of women but it is not legally allowed for rape, incest or physical deformities of the foetus. In 1999 the UN Human Rights Council recommended that Costa Rica (CR) should liberalize its law. However, this did not happen and it led to the refusal of the country to agree to an abortion for a 9-year-old girl who had suffered sex abuse. In the end she had a termination in Nicaragua. Doctors who suspect an abortion are required to report the fact to the Judicial Investigation Organization.

We have discussed the fact that misoprostol has created a safer abortion alternative. On 28 July 2008 an article was published: 'Costa Rican women can now buy abortion pills over the internet'. It continued to say that for 70 Euros a woman can access a website in one of seventy countries where the drug is available. However, another liberalizing move in 2008 met the wrath of the Government. This was an attempt by pro-choice groups to persuade women to use the morning after pill. The Government banned the attempt. (Hoffman 2008).

Although the anti-abortion forces in Costa Rica call themselves 'pro-life' they nevertheless oppose the use of IVF by women who would otherwise be infertile. This began in 2000 and when its Constitutional Court ruled that IVF was unconstitutional. This is discussed in the concluding chapter (Ertelt 2012).

Cuba

The population is 11.1 million (2013) and it is the most populated country in the Caribbean. Life expectancy from birth is 78.1 years. Its religion was at least 85 per cent Catholic before Castro came to power and promoted its variant of Marxist atheism. There is quite a strong Protestant minority with 300,000 members in 54 different denominations. In 1999 the Pope visited Cuba and publicly confronted Castro on the issue of religious freedom (Wright 2006, p. 563). In 2011 the birth rate was 9.9 per 1,000 and the death rate 7.6 per 1,000. This gives a rate of natural increase of 0.2 per cent. Its capital Havana had a population of 2.1 million in 2011 (CIA 2013, p. 186). Although the country pays lip service to Marxism, like the Soviet Union before, it does not follow his belief in the 'withering away of the state'; rather it has kept strong central control (Francome 2000). An example of this is that in 1983 Cuba destroyed all foreign blood products. During 1985 and beginning of 1986 it had a nationwide screening programme. The country has conducted over 20 million HIV tests and many people have been compulsorily detained (Barkside, accessed January 2014; d'Adesky, accessed January 2014) However, in 2011 Cuba had the lowest HIV prevalence in the Americas – 0.1 per cent – which was less than one tenth of the next lowest country (CIA 2013, p. 186). The country has specialized in medicine and has the second highest ratio of doctors to people in the world with only Italy having a higher proportion.

From 1870 until 1936 the abortion laws were those inherited from Spain. However, in the latter year there was liberalization and abortion was allowed on a range of grounds including to save the life or health of the woman, rape and abduction not followed by marriage. Abortions became available in private clinics (Babablu 2004). Abortion has been legal on request up until the tenth week of pregnancy since 1965. After that it is allowed for medical reasons (Acosta 2007). In 1986 there were 161,000 abortions registered. A 21-year-old student who had had two abortions commented 'something always gave, you either forgot one of the pills or the condom broke'. In 1996, 209,900 abortions were reported with a rate of 77.7 per 1,000 women 15–44 (Henshaw et al. 1999). However, the numbers began to fall until there were 67,300 in 2004 which is only one third of the figure eight years earlier. In part this is due to increasing use of menstrual regulation in the first six weeks of pregnancy. These are not recorded in the abortion figures and also do not require parental consent. In 2009 the figures rose to 85,000 despite the fact that 77 per cent of Cuban women of childbearing age used contraception (ETWN News 2011).

Ecuador

In 2013 the average woman had 2.3 children and the average length of life from birth was 76.2 years. The birthrate was 19.2 and death-rate was 5.0 giving a population growth rate of 1.4 per cent. The capital is Quito which had a population of 1.8 million in 2011. Its population is 95 per cent Catholic and five per cent other (CIA 2013, p. 213).

In 2012 the US group, Planned Parenthood, reported that the country had great instability and poverty – so much so that almost one in three of the population had no access to health care. It also pointed to figures showing that one third of pregnant women did not want to be so.

Planned Parenthood cooperated with the local organization CEMOPLAF which had been in operation for ten years spreading contraceptive information and were working in seventeen sites. In 2007 the two organizations launched an educational project for the Chimborag province where there had been a great amount of unwanted teenage pregnancy and a cycle of deprivation (Planned Parenthood 2012)

In 2008 in another example of co-operation the Dutch group, Women on Waves (WOW) received an invitation from the Ecuadorean Committee for Gender Equality to work together to set up an information hotline on safe abortion by means of misoprostol. At the launch it was reported:

> A banner was unfurled from the Virgin of del Parecillo, a statue of the virgin on a strategic hillside visible from most of Quito … the enormous banner reading 'Abortus Seguro 099004545' and a side banner read 'tu decision'. (Bloom 2008)

The relatively new availability has led to another dimension. The WOW website says to women 'Living in a country where safe abortion in not available? Get abortion pills online' (WOW 2012). So it seems that abortions will continue and be safer than hitherto.

In the light of this, the anti-abortion groups seem to be facing a difficult situation and have not considered this great change. In June 2012 Amparo Medina, the president of the Life and Family Network argued against any change in the law, for example, to allow abortion for rape. She commented 'A government that offers an abortion to a woman who has been raped as a solution to her problems shows how poor its social and human policies are' (Medina 2012).

El Salvador

In 2013 the average woman had 2.0 children and the length of life from birth was 73.9 years. The birthrate was 17.1 and the death rate was 5.7 giving a population growth rate of 1.1 per cent. The capital is San Salvador which had a population of 1.6 million in 2011. Its population is 57 per cent Catholic, 22 per cent various Protestant groups and 17 per cent no religion (CIA 2013, p. 221).

A civil war in the country ended in 1993 and conservative and religious groups made 28 December the assigned Feast of the Holy Innocents a special day to remember the unborn. Two years later a left wing guerrilla force known by the initials FMLN promoted a variety of women's issues. There was concern with domestic violence and rape and an attempt to liberalize the abortion law. The aim was to allow it on a variety of grounds such as the mental health of the woman. Up until this time the Catholic leaders in the country had been fairly radical and supported liberation theology, for example. However, in 1995 Pope John Paul 11 appointed a conservative – Lacalle – as archbishop. He was, for example, a member of Opus Dei (Hitt 2006) Despite the high Catholic involvement there was still relatively high contraceptive use with 73 per cent of woman 15–49 being protected (Global Health Facts 2013).

In 1997 a highly restrictive bill was introduced which banned all abortions. One of its supporters was Julia de Cardenal of the so-called 'Yes to Life' foundation. She argued 'There does not exist any case in which the life of the mother would be in danger because technology has advanced so far'. In one newspaper report she was quoted as saying 'The devil, tireless Prince of lies has tried and will continue to try to change our laws in order to kill our babies'. The bill passed in 1997 and came into effect in April 1998 (Hitt 2006).

Some women have received very long sentences. In November 2012 Marta Blandon of IPAS Central America reported that 'Karina' a woman with three children, had a tubal ligation but nevertheless became pregnant and was found to be haemorrhaging due to unsafe abortion. She was denied access to a lawyer and was sentenced to thirty years in prison. After eight years IPAS managed to get her a case review and she was freed. Sill however, Blandon reported that around 600 women were under investigation or prosecuted for suspicion of abortion related crimes. (2012).

One problem for hospital doctors it what to do with an ectopic pregnancy which one hospital reported happened about a 100 times a year. At some stage during development the foetus will rupture the Fallopian tube. One doctor reported that they kept the women in hospital and waited until the foetus died at which point they could operate and save the woman's life.

Under the 1997 Act abortion practitioners such as doctors or administrators could be sent to prison for up to 12 years, while women could be sentenced for up to eight years. If a woman were passed viability she could be charged with aggravated homicide which could lead to prison for 30 to 50 years. The local police took a very active role in prosecuting people and doctors were encouraged to break patient confidentiality and report abortion cases. From the laws inception until 20 August 2012, 628 women had been imprisoned accused of having a pregnancy termination (CAWN 2012).

A journalist interviewed a woman 'DC' who talked about her illegal abortion. She had a 7-year-old son and was four months pregnant. She went to a female practitioner who introduced a sound into her womb. She became ill and had to go to hospital and gave the practitioner's name to escape prison.

Observers suggest that there were three ways women obtained their abortions. The rich would go to Miami where they could have safe abortions under US law. The poor would get an illegal operator. The middle group would use a variety of methods. Most women would learn about misoprostol (Cytotec). If they took this they could go to hospital if they started bleeding. There was some risk of discovery 'if a doctor or nurse finds a half dissolved pill during a pelvic exam, then they are obliged to call the police.

The high level of reportage risks false accusations. One such was the case of a woman called Manuela who was a 32-year-old mother of two children. She had a miscarriage with severe complications and was in distress and went to the hospital. A doctor accused her of an illegal abortion and called the police. She was refused proper legal advice and was sentenced to 30 years imprisonment. Shortly after her incarceration she was diagnosed with advanced Hodgkin's Lymphoma which observers suggested could have been the cause of her emergency. In 2010 she died while still in prison (International Campaign, 27 September 2012).

Another innocent woman found guilty was Sonia Tabora. She had a miscarriage at seven months and a doctor thought that she had aborted herself. She was sentenced to 30 years in prison. However, campaigning led by the Citizen's Group for the Decriminalization of Abortion led to the authorities releasing her seven years into her sentence (CAWN 2012).

In July 2010, the 11th Regional Conference on women in Latin America and the Caribbean agreed to work to liberalize laws. The Catholic News Agency (CNA) reported complaints about the UN pressurizing El Salvador in this direction. It wanted the country to 'take measure to prevent women who seek treatment in public hospitals from being reported by health care workers or administrators for the crime of abortion' (CNA 2011). In 2012 the persecution of vulnerable women continued and the NY Centre for Reproductive Rights asked the Inter American Commission on Human Rights to intervene when El Salvador sent a woman to prison for two years for inducting an abortion (*Bloomsbury News* 2012).

Guatemala

In 2013 the average woman had 3.8 children which is high for the region. Its life expectancy at birth was 71.5 years. In that year too the birth rate was 26.0 per 1,000 and the death rate 4.9 per 1,000. This gives a rate of natural increase of 2.1 per cent. Its capital Guatemala City has a population of 1.1 million (2009 est.) (CIA 2013, p. 300).

In 1973 the law which had banned all abortions was slightly liberalized to allow the saving of a woman's life. This was despite the constitution stating the foetus had the right to life even from the moment of conception. In fact some Catholics believe abortion should never be carried out. For example Cardinal Rodolfo Q. Toruno said 'It is just as serious to kill a 10-year-old child or a 20-year-old adult as it is to kill a baby in his mother's womb (Westen 2008).

In 2003 a quality piece of research surveyed all the hospitals in Guatemala which treated post-abortion complications and also 74 professionals who were knowledgeable of local practice. It estimated that 65,000 illegal abortions were carried out each year which was around 24 per 1,000 women aged 15–49 (which is about 27 or 28 per 1,000 women aged 15–45). Around 32 per cent of pregnancies were unplanned (Singh 2006). Five years after this study it was still reported that illegal abortions were being carried out and was the leading cause of death amongst young women. A short film showed that one woman who died had used a corrosive liquid. It also drew attention to the importance of midwives in the local community in spreading family planning and so reducing the demand for abortion (Birthright 2011).

The drug Misoprostol will help reduce the country's problems with unsafe abortion. In 2011 over 100 women were introduced to the drug for an incomplete miscarriage with generally positive effects (Gynuity 2012). However, it does seem that gynaecologists are not up to date with medical abortion and study of 172 practitioners found that only 35 per cent knew the dosage for misoprostol recommended by the WHO and only 25 per cent knew about mifepristone. (Kestler 2012).

Guyana

The country gained its independence from the UK in 1966. In 2013 the average woman had 2.2 children and the length of life from birth was 67.7 years. In 2013 the birth rate was 16.3 births per 1,000 population and outstripped the death rate of 7.2. Nevertheless the population declined by 0.2 per cent presumably due to emigration. Its religion is 57 per cent Christian of which eight per cent are Catholic: Nearly three in ten (28 per cent) are Hindu due in large part to the past migration of Indian people to work on sugar plantations. Seven per cent were Muslim. Its capital is Georgetown with a population of 132,000 in 2009 (CIA 2013, p. 312).

The leading family planning organization is the Guyana Responsible Parenthood Association (GRPA). This was formed in 1974 and the IPPF reports that it is 'known across the country for free contraceptives'. In 2011 GRPA distributed 174,000 condoms as well as other activities. It is a member of the Caribbean Family Planning Affiliation (CFPA) (IPPF 2014). In discussing contraception we have drawn attention to the unmet need which is the percentage of fertile married women of reproductive age who do not wish to become pregnant but are not using contraception. This percentage declined from 32.4 per cent in 2007 to 28.5 per cent in 2009. This improvement nevertheless indicates there is still a great deal of room for improvement of usage (index mundi 2014). Guyana wants to increase contraceptive usage from 35 per cent to 60 per cent by 2020 by increasing the method mix and including long term methods and the integration of family [planning into the community services (IPPF 2014).

In 1991 septic abortion was the third leading cause of admittance to hospital and incomplete abortion was the eighth leading cause. In 1993 an intense public debate on changing the law began. In May 1993 Gail Teixeira, the Minister for Health and a strong supporter of liberalization. She described the abortion law as 'a law which no one cares to obey and no one dares to enforce' A committee of over thirty people was set up with people from a variety of places representing religious, legal, medical and feminist groups. This pro-reform group had as its main slogan 'Pro-life, Pro-Choice, Pro-Reform'. It sought to find common ground which was an unusual tactic (Nunes and Delph 1995). The aim of the law was said by a UN agency to be twofold. First, it was to improve health by reducing the number of unsafe abortions. Secondly it sought t to ;enhance the dignity of life by reducing the number of abortions' (UN 2014).

The new law – the Medical Termination of Pregnancy Act, was signed into law on 17 June 1995. It had different criteria according to gestation. In the first eight weeks abortion was legal if it were the wish of the woman and carried out by a qualified doctor or a person under his or her supervision in any setting. From 8 to 12 weeks it was legal if the abortion were carried out by a medical practitioner or a person under supervision in an approved institution. One of five conditions were also required. These were:

1. There was a likelihood of grave injury to the physical or mental health of the woman.
2. There was substantial risk that if born the child would be handicapped.
3. The woman believes the pregnancy was caused by rape or incest.
4. The woman was HIV positive.
5. The pregnancy was caused by contraceptive failure.

From 12–16 weeks it was legal if the woman had, in good faith, the approval of two doctors and met one of the five conditions above. Above 16 weeks there needed to be approval by three medical practitioners and meet certain conditions. These were to save the woman's life or prevent grave permanent injury to her health or to that of her child (UN 2014).

However, Nunes writing in 2012 said that 17 years after the liberal law was passed it was not being fully implemented and he gave an example of a young married mother of two, who died because of an unsafe abortion. She was only one year old when the law was passed yet still poor women could not get safe abortion in public hospitals.

Nunes points to one of the reasons for slow implementation in public hospitals was the removal of Gail Teixeira from the Ministry of Health. He pointed out that she 'clearly had a definite commitment to women's need for access to safe abortion.' Her successors did not have her zeal. Other factors such as lack of resources led Nunes to comment that the struggle for law reform is a short sprint whereas the implementation is like a marathon on a hot day on a course which only seems to go uphill. One of the bright spots is the work of the FPA of Guyana which has taught many doctors about manual vacuum aspiration and has been very successful with post-abortion contraception counselling having nearly a 100 per cent take up rate. Fred Nunes suggested in 1996 that if you calculate the number of women having their first abortion then the rate rose to show that 720 out of a 1,000 women had an abortion by the age of 45. This is a high incidence which will no doubt come down as contraception improves.

Haiti

In 2013 the average woman had 2.9 children and the length of life from birth was 62.9. The UN reports that for women in 1995–2000 female life expectation at birth was 56.2 years this rose to 64.3 years by the year 2013 which is a substantial increase of eight years (UN Secretariat, accessed 16 January 2014, CIA 2013, p. 316). Four out of five (80 per cent) people are Catholic and one in six (16 per cent) Protestant. Observers report that roughly half the population practices voodoo. The capital city is Port-au-Prince with a population of 2.1 million in 2010 (CIA 2013, p. 317).

We have seen earlier in this chapter that the maternal mortality rate in Haiti is four times the median for Latin America and twice the median infant mortality rate.

Health Ministry officials say post-abortion complications now account for as many as 30 per cent of maternal deaths on the island (Martin 2013).

Women seem to have great problems in accessing modern methods of contraception. In the period 1994–95 only 13 per cent of married women used modern contraceptives. This increased to one third (32 per cent) on the period 2005–2010 (Global Health Facts 2013). A Government sponsored survey in 2013 showed a great gap between what women wanted and what they could access. Over a third (35 per cent) of married women in the age range 15–49 stated that they would like to control the number of their children or at least to regulate births but did not have access to contraception. This is despite the fact that contraception is provided free by the UN Population Fund (Charles 2013). There does seem to be increasing concern about birth control from those in positions of power. So in 2013 the country's President Michel Martelly issued a presidential decree calling upon all state institutions to provide counselling and free contraception (Charles 2013).

As far as the issue of abortion is concerned the Haiti law is based on the French Penal Code of 1810. Strictly speaking, the law bans abortion on all grounds. However, the UN states that in practice abortions can be obtained for rape, physical health of the woman, incest and foetal abnormality (UN Secretariat, accessed 16 January 2014). As always, rich women can become abortion 'tourists'. An Indian hospital – Bangalore Genesis – placed an advertisement in Haiti which commented on the situation in the country. 'The best method of abortion for women living in Haiti is simply to leave the country' (Advertisement 2014).

In January 2010 a massive earthquake (7.0) struck Haiti with its epicentre about 15 miles west of the capital. Estimates were that 300,000 people were killed and 1.5 million made homeless which is above 15 per cent of the population. The earthquake was assessed as the worst in the region for the previous 200 years (CIA 2013, p. 316). In the transcript of a television interview Jacqueline Charles reported some of the ramifications of the earthquake on fertility (December 2013):

> Medical aid groups started to notice with the explosion of the tent babies that there were a lot of women who were suffering from post-abortion complications. After the earthquake there was an explosion of tent cities that took place around

> the capital and the cities in surrounding areas. There was a high fertility rate that was happening in these tent cities. Some of it was voluntary, some of it was because it was survival, and some of it was because it was rape.
>
> It's really tragic because what happens is that someone with money can go to a private doctor and they can secretly get an abortion with anesthesia and in a sterilized environment. When you talk to young girls they turn to herbal concoctions. They turn to the pill that is really an anti-ulcer drug but it's readily available on the street of Haiti or at any pharmacy without a prescription. (Charles 2013)

She continued to say that many people did not know how to use the pill and consequently faced haemorrhaging and infection. Charles also related the 'heartbreaking' story of a young girl who had nearly finished school. She did not want to tell her parents and so sought outside help:

> First she went to a clinic and they inserted some instrument in her and perforated her uterus. That did not work. She was four months pregnant. Then she went to a herbal doctor … He give her some special bath using all these different concoctions, including Haiti moonshine. (Charles 2013)

This led her to abort, however, it was incomplete. She was very ill for three days and then went to a 'doctor's without borders' hospital. This repaired her uterus, however, she was in hospital for two months and when interviewed was very weak (Charles 2013).

In 2013 there were signs of a wish to help and the health ministry brought together religious leaders, women's groups, doctors and social workers and said that they needed to address the issue and draft a law that could be presented to Parliament. So with positive signs from the president there could be moves to improve the social support and aid women's health (Charles 2013).

Honduras

In 2013 the average woman had 2.9 children and its life expectancy at birth was 70.8 years. Its religion is 97.0 per cent Catholic and three per cent Protestant. In the year 2013 the birth rate was 24.2 per 1,000 and the death rate 5.0 per 1,000 (2011). This gives a rate of natural increase of 1.9 per cent. Its capital Tegucigalpa has a population of one million (2009 est.) (CIA 2012, p. 291 and CIA 2013, p. 322).

In the years 2005–2010 the 65 per cent of women in relationships aged 15–49 were using contraceptives. This is slightly higher than the world average (WHO 2012).

The penal code of 1906 had no exceptions from an overall prohibition on abortion. However, in 1964 abortion was legalized to save the life of the woman.

In 1983 the legislature passed a law to legalize abortion for rape, incest and foetal problems. At the International Conference on Population and Development at Cairo in 1994 the representatives from Honduras explained its position. This was that they accepted family planning, reproductive health statements and measures to reduce maternal mortality.

In 1984 there was a pastoral declaration of the Honduras Bishop's Conference (3 May). This opposed the use of abortion for rape. It commented 'a wrong perpetuated against the woman victimized by rape cannot be erased by a worse action.'

One unusual development was a moral panic over post-coital contraception. In 2009 the Catholic News Agency reported that the Congress in Honduras prohibits the 'morning after pill'. One argument was that 'It has been shown to be an abortifacient and very harmful to the youth'. In 2012 a commentator noted the 'Honduras Supreme Court upholds the most sweeping ban on emergency contraception anywhere' (Jacobson 2012).

This led to a critic saying 'Honduras is telling the world it would rather imprison the women of its country than provide them with safe and effective birth control. The president took a different view and gave a green light to the 'morning after' pill (Catholic News Agency 2009).

Jamaica

In 2013 the average woman had 2.1 children which is just around replacement level. The length of life from birth was 73.4. The birth rate was 18.7 per 1,000 and the death rate was 6.6. This gives a rate of increase of 1.2 per cent. Its capital Kingston had a population of 580,000 in 2009 (CIA 2013, p. 369).

In 1864 the country had inherited the UK's restricted and unclear Offences against the Person Act (1861) which led to a well-developed illegal abortion network. This was considered when in 2005 the decision was taken to review the abortion law. An advisory group was set up. It carried out a six-month study and found that the high number of women having to go to hospital because of the effects of unsafe abortion was leading to pressure on public health centres. It commented that the women seeking abortion were 'young, poor, unemployed and live in economically and social deprived communities'. It was recommended that a liberalization of the law take place but there was no change (Gabbatt 2012).

On 6 May 2012 a substantial newspaper report appeared in the *Gleaner* entitled 'Abortion for sale – black market thrives on baby killing pills'. It reported that a local health professional was selling misoprostol without prescription. The *Gleaner* decided to carry out its own research and found the drug was very easy to buy. The instructions suggested the woman should ingest two pills and then introduce three high up in the vagina one at a time. Its report was very much opposed to the use of the pills. However, it quoted a Dr Horace Fletcher who said that misoprostol had led to a reduction in hospital visits as women no longer had to go to 'unscrupulous persons who would insert unclean objects and cause sepsis (*Gleaner* 2012).

In July 2012 an award winning Jamaican doctor – Lloyd Goldson – was arrested by the police for performing an abortion on a 12-year-old girl at the request of her mother who was also arrested. The facts came to police attention when the girl suffered minor complications and attended hospital. The case has caused a great deal of controversy and reports quoted the head of the FPA in Barbados as saying 'In no circumstances should 11- or 12-year-olds be allowed to carry pregnancies to term (Gabbat 2012). The situation has not been resolved as far as we can tell (February 2014).

Mexico

In 2013 the average woman had 2.3 children. It used to be much higher and for example was 5.6 children per woman in 1976 (Durabi). The life expectancy at birth was 76.9 years. The birth rate was 18.6 per 1,000 and the death rate 4.9 per 1,000. This gives a rate of natural increase of 1.4 per cent. Mexico has a federal policy and consists of 31 states and the Federal District. Its religion is 83 per cent Catholic and ten per cent Protestant. Its capital is Mexico City which in 2009 had a population of 19.3 million (CIA 2013, p. 479).

Research by the Population Council of Mexico and the Guttmacher Institute in NY stated that the number of abortions in Mexico rose from 533,000 in 1990 to 875,000 in 2006. This is a rate of 33 per thousand women aged 15–45 years which is over 50 per cent more than the US figure. This led the lead author to comment 'Making abortion illegal does not significantly reduce its frequency, it just makes it unsafe and puts women's lives at risk'. (Juarez et al. 2008).

Contraceptive use increased from below three in five (58 per cent) married and cohabiting women in 1990 to three quarters (75 per cent) in the year 2,000 and of these (66 per cent) were using modern methods of contraception (UN 2004, p. 57). Female sterilization grew from nine per cent of married women in 1976 to 36 per cent in 1987 (del Carmen Elu 1993). If this change had not occurred the abortion rate would have been even higher.

Abortion had been a crime since 1931. It had exceptions for the life of the woman, rape and the curious situation 'where the abortion is the result of negligent behaviour of the pregnant woman'. Another curiosity of the Mexican law was that there was a lower penalty for abortion with a maximum sentence of one year for a woman 'who does not have a bad reputation' (Human Rights Watch 2007d). A major change occurred in April 2007 when Mexico City decided to make abortion legal on request in the first trimester and was the first Latin American area to take this decision outside Cuba. This was confirmed in the following year when the Supreme Court ruled that there was no legal impediment to abortion.

Illegal abortion has been common for some time. In 1989 the police stormed an abortion clinic and detained eight women with a resultant series of protests (del Carmen 1993). In 1991 in Mexico City observers report one in two of the pregnant women hospitalized were there through unsafe abortion (del Carmen Elu1993). The fact that abortion is cheaper in Mexico has meant that some US women travelled there for their abortion. Financial support was denied to poor US women during the Presidency of Jimmy Carter. Feminists in the US were very angry about the decision and especially so when a woman died in Mexico. A book entitled 'Rosie' was written about her.

Although abortion was legal for rape it has often proved difficult for women to obtain. A major report on the issue told of one 13-year-old girl – pregnant by a family member – who was made to watch a factually inaccurate film by a social worker. Others had had their abortion denied. In one such case a 16-year-old was raped weekly by her father. She said in her evidence: (Human Rights Watch 2006d).

> Then my father took me to a hostel. He penetrated me and it hurt a lot when he penetrated me. I cried and I said to my father that it hurt a lot. I want to declare that I don't want to have the child I am expecting, because I won't be able to love it because it is my father's.

This led to Kenneth Roth of Human Rights Watch commenting 'Pregnant rape victims are essentially assaulted twice – first by the perpetrators who rape them and then by the public figures that ignore them, insult them and deny them a legal abortion'.

The decision of Mexico City to decriminalize abortion in the first trimester seems to have galvanized the conservatives. Maria Mejia of the group Catholics for the Right to Decide said there was pact between conservative groups and the Catholic church. Both she and Maria L Sanchez of the Information Group on Reproductive Health (GIRE) called for the decriminalization of abortion (*Huffington Post* 2009).

It seems that abortion is far more problematical in Mexico than elsewhere. For example 17 per cent of Mexican women needed to go to hospital after an abortion compared to only 0.3 per cent in the US (Darabi 2012). There is one organization GIRE which is openly in favour of a Women's Right to Choose and other pressure groups in addition to the Mexican chapter of Catholics for a Free Choice. These could have a greater effect in future years (Illingworth 2006).

Panama

In July 2013 its life expectancy at birth was 78.1 years and the average woman had 2.4 children. This is a substantial reduction from 6.0 in 1965 and 3.0 in 1985 (UN, accessed January 2004) Its religion is 85 per cent Catholic and 15 per cent Protestant. In the year 2013 the birth rate was 18.9 per 1,000 and the death rate 4.7

per 1,000. This gives a rate of natural increase of 1.4 per cent. Its capital Panama City has a population of 1.3 million (2009 est.) (CIA 2013, p. 561).

Panama differs from much of the rest of the continent in that while it opposes abortion it holds a positive view of family planning. In 1965 it set up its local family planning organization in conjunction with outside organizations from the US. It has continued the support and provides free condoms and the pill. It also supplies relatively cheap injectable contraception and permits sterilization for women who have had at least three children. However, women need to obtain their husband's permission. In 1973 The Government began providing subsidies for contraception.

In contrast, the country is very much opposed to abortion. In 2005 an opinion poll asked the question 'Do you agree or disagree with abortion'. In response 89.4 per cent replied that they did not. Although this does not mean that all these people support an abortion ban. It is perfectly reasonable for people to say that while they personally do not agree with abortion they do not wish to interfere with people's choice. The law in Panama was relatively strict with women who aborted being given one to three years in prison and longer sentences for doctors performing the operations (PRI 2006).

In 2006 several observers said that Panama was very much a pro-life country. They claimed, for example, that there were no abortions in Panama except under carefully specified procedures for the sake of the woman and continued to say that the presence of good quality contraception meant that the number of illegal abortions were relatively few. Also the organization APLAFA (Association Panamena parael Planeamiento de la Familia) provided help to pregnant women with problems. A few women may well travel abroad – especially to Florida. However, overall the article talked of there being a 'gratifying pro-life picture' (PRI 2006).

Despite this optimism that women would not need abortions a few years later the number of illegal abortions had grown to such a degree that in 2012 there were demonstrations by anti-abortion groups which were protesting the high number of operations (Anderson 2012). A fractious debate seems likely and that women will continue to be unable to access safe legal abortions.

Peru

In 2013 the average woman had 2.2 children which is just above replacement level. Life expectancy at birth was 73.0 years. Its religion is 81 per cent Catholic. In 2013 the birth rate was 18.9 per 1,000 and the death rate 6.0 per 1,000. This gives a rate of natural increase of 1.3 per cent. Its capital city Lima had a population of 8.8 million in 2099 (CIA 2013, p. 572).

Contraceptive use increased from over half (54 per cent) married and cohabiting women in 1990 to seven out of ten (69 per cent) in the year 2,000 and of these half (50 per cent) were using modern methods of contraception (UN 2004,

p. 57). During the period 2005–2010 the percentage of women using modern contraception increased to 73.2 per cent. This figure is higher than rich countries like the Netherlands (69.0 per cent) and Spain (65.7 per cent). It would have clearly led to fewer abortions than otherwise (Global Health Facts 2013, p. 3).

The abortion law in Peru allows the operation to save the woman's life and in order to protect the woman's physical and mental health. However, some of the interpretations of the law have come under criticism. In one case 'KL' a 17-year-old woman went for a scan and anencephaly was diagnosed. Despite the fact that this condition is fatal for the foetus she was denied an abortion and was forced to care for the baby for the four days until it died. The case resulting from this event led to it being the first one for the United Nations Human Rights Committee. It ruled that the Government 'in denying access to legal abortion violates a woman's basic human rights'. This was the first time that an international human rights body had held a Government responsible for failing to secure access to a legal abortion. *The New York Times* carried the story (17 November 2005) under the headline 'Woman forced to carry fatally impaired foetus to term wins case'. Luisa Cabal commented on the case.

> Every woman who lives in any of the 154 countries that are part of this treaty – including the US – now has a legal tool to use in defense of her rights. When abortion is legal it is the government's duty to ensure that women have access to it'.

The article continued to say that in Peru there are 85,000 women who are sexually active, of reproductive age, who do not want children and yet have no access to contraception. This is a quarter of all women in this group.

In 2007 it was estimated that there were 410,000 unsafe abortions every year (International Women's Health Coalition 2007). Human rights groups produce a slightly lower figure of 370,000 abortions in 2009 (BBC 2009). One observer commented on the situation 'Clandestine abortion continues to be one of the main ways women control their health'.

One of the organizations working in Peru is Pathfinder International (PI) which has won some useful concessions. These enabled it to improve after-care in the case of unsafe abortions and to provide contraceptive advice after birth or abortion (Webb 2000). One of the parts of its programme is to promote MVA. It arranged training for doctors and nurses and found it was more effective that dilation and curettage for after abortion care. In Peru the cost of a D&C is four times that of MVA. Furthermore PI reported that nurses commented that the training had created an atmosphere in which they were no longer afraid to display empathy towards the patient. PI worked in hand with the Government of Peru trained doctors and nurses in post-abortion aftercare with MVA (Webb 2000).

In 2007 Milka Dinev and colleagues reported that in 2005–2006, 1565 women attending for an abortion were offered either two 800ml doses of misoprostol separated by 24 hours or MVA. A total of 812 chose the medical abortion option and 753 MVA. The medical option was 80 per cent successful and when it did not work MVA was provided. Dinev and colleagues commented 'High quality service can be provided in countries with restrictive laws.'

There has been other activity for change in Peru. In 2009 the BBC reported 'clashes over Peru abortion move'. Its correspondent Dan Collyus commented that 'passions are rising high'. This was because of plans to introduce a liberalizing bill which would allow a legal termination for rape, incest or foetal deformity. Lisette Roman was quoted as saying that women were dying every day whilst getting clandestine abortions'.

Another case led to UN action. A 13-year-old girl became pregnant after rape and decided to commit suicide by jumping off a building. The attempt failed and fractured her spine. The evidence suggests that the damage could have been repaired, but the doctors refused to treat her in case they damaged the foetus. She subsequently miscarried and received treatment but it was too late to prevent her being severely disabled. The Centre for Reproductive rights (CRR) was one of the organizations bringing legal action which led to the UN action and to a CRR press release (2011) Part of it read

> The UN Committee for the Elimination of Discrimination Against Women (CEDAW) ruled Peru must amend its law to allow women to obtain an abortion in the case of rape and sexual assault and establish a mechanism to ensure the availability of those abortion facilities and guarantee access to abortion facilities when a woman's life or health is in danger. (CRR 2011)

However, Catholic News Agency (CNA) reported that several abortion opponents said the ruling was not binding and it was not implemented (CNA 2013) This is problematical for the women of Peru for the country has the highest rate of rape and sexual violence in the South America and one estimate is that there are 35,000 women pregnant by rape each year (Girard 2012). So the current situation produces a great deal of suffering for the local women.

Puerto Rico

The 2013 figures show the country has a birthrate which is below replacement level at 1.6 children per woman. Its length of life is 79.1 years. Its religion is 85 per cent Catholic and fifteen per cent Protestant and other (CIA 2013, p. 589). In 2913 the birth rate was 11.3 per 1,000 and the death rate 8.2 per 1,000. This gives a rate of natural increase of 0.3 per cent which is half what it was eight years earlier. Its capital city is San Juan with a population of 2.7 million in 2009 (CIA 2013, p. 589). Puerto Rico is an autonomous political entity in voluntary association with the US. Its constitution came in to effect on 22 July 1952 when it changed from being a US colony. Its political structure is modelled on that of the US and it too celebrates US Independence Day (4 July). Contraceptive services in the country date back to 1925 when Dr Jose Rolon had contacts with the US activist Margaret Sanger, who in turn had close links with the British proponents (Francome 1984, p. 61). One of the aims was to reduce the incidence of illegal abortion. The first clinic was opened in the city of Ponce and several more followed until in the 1930s they were briefly closed after pressure from the Catholic Church which opposed both contraception and abortion. In the 1950s the pill was first tested in Puerto Rico before it was legalized in the United States and Britain. Historically, there have been strong sex divisions with men being expected to express machismo and women to play the subservient role. Maria is by far the most common name and in some families more that one daughter might even be so named with an alternative as a second name. This is to remind women of the Virgin Mary and her acceptance of her lot. A perhaps surprising finding by numerous researchers is that Catholics use contraception and abortion just as much as non-Catholics (Montesmos and Precido 2007).

The mere fact that abortion is legal in Puerto Rico is not enough if the Government, NGOs, doctors, universities and other health-based organizations are not involved in the process of educating and informing the general public about the issue. Some of the barriers to accessing safe abortion services in Puerto Rico include: a lack of information on its legal status, a shortage of skilled and available providers, the high cost of the services, stigmatization, by moral or religious values, and the fact that only nine clinics are certified. A primary limitation is that most service providers require the presence of an adult. For young women, cost is also one of the major barriers to access. Moreover, seven of the nine public clinics that currently offer abortion services are in the metropolitan area, limiting access to women in rural areas or in other areas of the country. The other two clinics are in the southern and northwestern parts of the country.

In 2012 there was some debate over abortion and five women appeared on a radio programme. There were complaints from women activists and one was quoted in the media as saying 'The State cannot impose a single morality on the diversity of thoughts and beliefs. Women decide what to do with their own bodies, sex and lives' (International Campaign 2013).

Trinidad and Tobago

In 2013 the average woman had 1.7 children which is below replacement level. Life expectancy at birth was 72.0 years. Its religion was 26 per cent Catholic, 32 per cent Protestant and 22 per cent Hindu. Also in the year 2013 the birth rate was 14.3 per 1,000 and the death rate 8.4 per 1,000. This gives a rate of natural increase of 0.6 per cent despite the fact that in the longer term the low number of births will lead to a reduction in population size unless there is significant immigration. Its capital, Port of Spain has a population 57,000 (2009 estimate) (CIA 2012, p. 735).

Economy relies on income from gas and oil. It also is involved in drugs which make up around three per cent of its GNP.

Trinidad and Tobago are just seven kilometres from Venezuela. Abortion is largely illegal but is allowed to save the life of the woman. Any doctor or woman involved in a abortion risks being sent to prison for up to four years.

In 2001, the organization entitled 'Advocates for Safe Parenthood Improving Reproductive Equity (ASPIRE)' was formed. This pro-choice organization aimed to improve the health of women by mitigating the effects of unsafe abortions. In 2007 a poll showed that around half the population wanted improved access to abortion (Kowlesser 2012). One of the problems is that in the period 2005–2010 only 43 per cent of women (15–49 used any method of contraception. (WHO 2012). It is therefore not surprising that the abortion rate is relatively high. The Caribbean Catholic reported in May 2012 that the abortion rate was 45 per 1,000 women of childbearing age. This it compared to a rate of 27 in the US (Caribbean Catholic 2012).

In 2012 the politician Verna St Rose Greaves called for abortion to be legalized. A crucial factor was that each year over 4,000 women were hospitalized. The health minister Fuad Khan responded by saying that many women died from 'backyard abortions'. Others suffered from infertility.

A heartrending case was of a 11-year-old girl who was raped and made pregnant by her father. Although abortion for rape is not legal there was a great deal of concern about her physical health and the fact that such a young body is not ready for the rigours of labour. One commentator stated: 'How will she survive bringing up a child, going to school, growing up and leading a normal life' (Kissoon 2012).

Uruguay

In 2013 the average woman had 1.9 children which is below replacement level. Its life expectancy at birth was 76.6 years. Its religion is almost half Catholic (47 per cent), Just over a third (34 per cent) are Protestant, almost one in five (17 per cent) are agnostic or atheist and 0.3 per cent Jewish. Less than half the population attends worship regularly (CIA 2013, p. 776). Its capital city is Montevideo with a population of 1.6 million in 2009. In the 1970s the country was under a military regime and was reported to have the highest ratio of political prisoners in Latin America.

Abortion was made illegal in 1938 and a commentator said about the decision, 'The abortion law was not the result of serious debate but of trivial discussion while approving the national budget for the year' (Choike 2002). There was an unusual feature of the law in Uruguay in that 'No economic or social justification make an abortion legal but when such a defence is offered, the penalty for breaking the law is waived'. There is also the provision that an abortion can be allowed in case of 'jeopardy of a man's honour' (Choike 2002). When military rule ended there were numerous attempts to liberalize the law. One such attempt in 2002 led to a bill being approved by the House of Representatives in December by 47 votes to 40 with 10 representatives not voting. However, the Senate blocked the legislation. It faced great opposition from the Catholic Church which read out the names of those voting for the Act at mass. Furthermore, five Republicans from the US led by Chris Smith sent faxes to the Senators urging them to oppose the Act. The Methodists were more supportive and on 11 February 2003 the Evangelical Methodist Church of Uruguay published a statement on abortion which stated:

> The Methodist church does not condone abortion or anything else that attacks human life. However, we must not fall into the trap of confusing decriminalization with inciting or promoting abortion.

It continued to say that there would be two positive factors to come out of a liberalization of the law. The first is that it would clearly improve the overall health of women who would not have to face illegal operations and secondly it would help to reduce discrimination against women

In the end it failed. However, in 2004 a relaxation occurred when the Ministry of Public Health approved a measure which allows doctors to give advice to women who want abortions. It hoped that this change would result in a reduction in problems from unsafe abortions. Gara Bossio, who took the post of Chief Justice of Uruguay's Supreme Court, made it clear that she wanted change. In particular she said she was worried about poor women 'They have many kids and have no way to obtain abortions, while women who are well off can go to any clinic and get one'. (CAN/LW News 2007). Reports stated that there would be an attempt to bring in abortion on request.

An estimate relating to 2002 was that each year there were 30,000–50,000 abortions. Until legalization unsafe abortions will continue. In 2004 the New Internationalist reported that abortion caused 47 per cent of the maternal deaths at the leading maternity hospital (Pereira Rossell) compared to 28 per cent in the rest of the country:

> Flavia was 16 and had a six-month-old baby that she was still breastfeeding at night. She had no access to sex education or abortion clinics and only an abortion pill that she put in her vagina. Rosario Echargue was the doctor who received her at the hospital an hour after she had used the pill 'She had a pain in her stomach abundant diarrhoea and unstoppable vomiting. She was pale and trembling, did not understand what was happening to her. She died and she was not even pregnant. (Fonseca and Pujol 2004)

IPPF states that there is an estimate that for each death due to unsafe abortion, there are 10 women with complications and 100 with minimum consequences. In addition Senator A Couriel stated that for every death there are many women whose condition is so dire that they will never have a child. This concern with unsafe abortion continued. And before legalization a dozen women appeared nude in a demonstration against the law. They braved cold weather and had their bodies painted orange with purple flowers (International Campaign 2012b).

Activists also pointed to the fact that they had public support. In September 2012, the Lower House voted to legalize abortion by the razor-thin margin of 50–49. On 17 October it passed through the Senate by 17–14 votes. The bill did not fulfil the all the wishes of feminist groups because it had a number of restrictions. Its main features were as follows:

- Women should have the right to a legal abortion for the first 12 weeks of pregnancy.
- Women suffering rape should be able to obtain an abortion until 14 weeks.
- Later, abortions were legal if the foetus was predicted not to be able to survive at birth.
- Women must go before a panel of three to listen to advice for example about support services available.
- There was a five-day waiting period for women to reflect on the decision.
- There was a residential requirement that women had live in the country for a year.

A local activist was upset by all the restrictions and commented. 'This is not the law for which we fought for more than 25 years, In the Senate, passage of the bill was easier (BBC 2012).

Lawmaker Luis Gallo commented that this change of law helped put Uruguay on a par with the rich countries which had already legalized the operation.

There was an attempt by anti-abortion forces to get enough support to have a referendum on the issue. In the event 655,000 votes were needed but only around a third of this figure (226,653 votes) were collected. Consequently, the Act will continue to stand.

Venezuela

In 2013 the average woman had 2.4 children. This is higher than many in the region. However, there has been over a 50 per cent reduction from 5.9 children per woman in 1970. In 2013, life expectancy at birth was 74.2 years. Its religion is nominally 96 per cent Catholic and two per cent Protestant. In the year 2013 the birth rate was 19.7 per 1,000 and the death rate 5.2 per 1,000. This gives a rate of natural increase of 1.5 per cent. Its capital city is Caracas with a population of 3.1 million (2009) (CIA 2013, p. 787).

Under the Criminal code of 1964, abortion is illegal in Venezuela except to save the life of the woman. Legal abortion needs the written consent of the woman, her husband or a legal representative. In 1986 there was a proposal for reform to permit abortion on therapeutic grounds such as the woman's physical or mental health or rape, incest and eugenics. However, this law has not yet been incorporated. In 2005 supporters of President Hugo Chavez unsuccessfully lobbied for abortion on the grounds of rape and incest (UN Population Committee 2007).

In 2011 it was estimated that each year 50–100 women died of illegal abortion and a further 500–1,000 were hospitalized (Population Policy 2011). This was estimated to have been a reduction and seems largely to be due to the decline in demand for abortion because of improved birth control. It may also reflect improved treatment. The Government believes that the abortion problem 'can be alleviated by the increased provisions of family life education and family planning services'. The Government has also created the ministry of the family which was the first institution of its kind in Latin America.

In May 2011 there was an important development when a 'safe abortion hotline' was set in Caracas. It said 'Women in Venezuela call 0246–1169496'. The idea was that women would be told how to carry out safe abortions with misoprostol. WOW was closely involved and the organizers had help from Ecuadorian feminists. The hotline aimed not only to help women but also to raise awareness (WOW 2012).

Conclusion

The evidence of Latin America shows strongly the effect of the Catholic Church with many countries showing evidence of lack of modern contraception and abortion laws that are very restrictive. We have seen some surprising differences between countries. The moral panic in Honduras over post-coital contraception is one illustration, The surprising arrest of a gynaecologist in Jamaica for carrying out an abortion on a 12-year-old girl is also unexpected. This is especially the case as the country generally follows British law which legalized abortion for rape in 1938 (Francome 1984, p. 69).

The evidence shows that there is a relationship in that those countries with legal abortion have fewer unsafe abortions and health problems for women in comparison with those where abortion is only allowed on restricted grounds.

The change in the Law in Mexico City could have important and long lasting effects. Furthermore, the advent of medical abortion and greater access of MVA could have an important influence on future developments.

One of the differences between Latin America and European countries is that the liberalization of abortion in Europe is more linked to the Left wing. If this applied to Latin America we might have expected more change. Local observers commented that over the 10 years to 2012 there has been a move to more progressive parties with 11 being more radical. These are Argentina, Bolivia, Brazil, Chile, Cuba, Ecuador, El Salvador, Nicaragua, Paraguay, Uruguay and Venezuela. Six are more to the Right: Columbia, Costa Rica, Honduras, Mexico, Panama, and Peru; two are moderate: Guyana and Dominica.

At least three countries do not allow abortion to save a woman's life and all three are otherwise generally progressive: Chile, El Salvador and Nicaragua. None of the six right-wing countries rejected saving a woman's life.

The legalization in Mexico City did come from left-wing forces. It does seem that there might be number countries which may liberalize in the future.

There are a few bright spots on the horizon. The decision of the previous Pope in 2011 to approve of condoms is a major change. Although he originally did it for the health protection of male homosexuals it clearly has wider implications. For example if a husband is carrying the HIV virus it would be logical for the wife to be able to protect herself with a condom.

The introduction of MVA and misoprostol can work in the short term in reducing the harm from unsafe abortions. However, what is really needed is a widespread move towards giving women the right to choose. In this respect we might like to consider the position of the Massachusetts priest Father Drinan who took the view the Catholic Church should stay out of the debate (Francome 1984, pp. 203–4). Furthermore there is a case for saying that the former colonial powers for the continent including Spain, Portugal and the UK should help in whatever ways they can to enable Latin America and the Caribbean to enjoy the benefits of safe abortion as do their own women.

Chapter 6
Oceania

> 'Many people believe pregnancy will not occur until couples have sex at least six times'. (Oliver-Miller 2004)

The region had an abortion rate of 17 per 1,000 women aged 15–44 years which is well below the world average of 28. All but two of these abortions are safe.

Oceania's population growth has reduced in recent years. In the period 1970–75 it was 5.8 children per woman. It fell to 2.5 in the period 1990–5 and to 2.4 from 1995–2000 (UN 2004, p. 29).

Oceania includes both developed countries (Australia/New Zealand) and less developed areas *Melanesia/Micronesia/Polynesia*, which consists of Fiji, French Polynesia, Guam, New Caledonia, Papua New Guinea, Solomon Islands, Samoa, Timor Leste and Vanuatu).

Table 6.1 Oceania: maternal and infant mortality

	Maternal mortality rate (deaths per 100,000 live births)	Infant mortality rate (deaths per 1,000 live births)	Population millions
	2010	2013	2013
Australia	7	4.5	22.1
Fiji	26	10.7	0.9
French Polynesia	n/a	4.8	0.3
Guam	n/a	5.6	0.2
New Caledonia	n/a	5.5	0.3
New Zealand	15	4.7	4.4
Papua New Guinea	230	40.8	6.4
Samoa	100	21.0	0.2
Solomon Islands	93	16.7	0.6
Timor Leste	300	40.1	1.2
Vanuatu	110	27.2	0.3

Source: CIA 2013, selected pages, pp. 41–785.

The table shows some wide differences in health, with the maternal mortality rate in Papua New Guinea and Timor Leste being of a different order to Australia and New Zealand. Timor Leste has over 40 times the maternal mortality rate of

Australia while Papua New Guinea has over 30 times the Australian rate. We will consider the four largest countries in the region in more detail and Vanuatu to provide variety.

Australia

Population was estimated at 22.1 million and life expectancy from birth at 81.9 years in 2011. Its religion (2006 Census) is 38 per cent Protestant, 26 per cent Catholic, two per cent Muslim and also Buddhist the other 32 per cent were unspecified or had no religion (CIA 2013, p. 41). In 2013 the birth rate was 12.2 per 1,000 and the death rate 7.0. This gives a rate of natural increase of 0.5 per cent. However, including immigration the growth rate is 1.1 per cent. In 2013 the average woman had 1.8 children (CIA 2013, p. 42). Its capital city is Canberra with a population of 384,000 but the two biggest cities are Sydney with 4.4 million and Melbourne 3.9 million (2009 estimates). Like the US, Australia has a federal structure. However, because there is no Supreme Court each of the states can decide its own law. There is the Capital Territory and seven states as follows: South Australia, Victoria, Northern Territory, Tasmania, New South Wales, Western Australia and Queensland. In 2013 the UN voted Australia as number one in the world in terms of quality of life (UN 2013).

The Australian FPA was formed in 1952 and has a great deal of government support. Staton reports that the government's family planning programme aims to reduce both maternal and infant mortality. It also aims to reduce the number of unwanted pregnancies and so the need for abortion (Staton 2013). In 2010 the major organizations celebrated 50 years of the contraceptive pill. On the 26 February 2013, the Queensland Senator Clair Moore gave an important speech to the Australian Senate. She said that although a great deal of progress had been made there were still challenges ahead in the area of reproduction. Australia for example has an annual teenage pregnancy rate of 16 per 1,000. This contrasts with five for Singapore and an average of six for Denmark and Sweden. She also drew attention to ethnic divisions. The latest infant mortality rate was 3.8 per 1,000 live births in 2011 but was 7.2 for aboriginal and Torres Strait Islands people (Moore 2013).

The Australian abortion laws were rooted in the 1861 British Act. As in some other countries such as the US, when activists began to think about liberalizing their laws they had to choose whether to work for change through parliament or to make legal challenges in the courts. Different states chose different paths. Before legalization, abortion was often performed by doctors for financial gain and with the agreement of the local police. Evidence for this came in 1969 in Victoria when four members of the police force were convicted after abortionists were offered protection against prosecution for ten per cent of their fees (Wainer 1972). This raised interest in the possibility of a change in the law as did the 1967 British Act. South Australia was the first state to pass a liberal law in 1969. The wording was akin to that in Britain and allowed abortion when 'continuance of the pregnancy would involve greater risk to the life of the pregnant woman or greater risk of injury to the physical or mental health of the pregnant woman than if the pregnancy were terminated'. This wording had been used to support abortion on request in Britain.

Victoria differed from South Australia in that the law was changed through the courts. It was broadened by the case *R* v *Davidson*, 1969, where a State Supreme Court Judge had to give direction on the use of the word 'unlawfully' as placed in the British 1861 Act and copied into the legislation. Later, in 2002, Victoria legalized abortion on request up to 24 weeks.

Northern Territory passed a liberalizing law in 1973 (Paxman 1980). It then gave women the right to choose up to 14 weeks, and later when there is a serious risk to the woman's health. In Tasmania from 1925 to 2001 the law prohibited 'unlawful abortion'. However, in 2001 it passed a law similar to that of Southern Australia. In 2013 Tasmania eliminated criminal sanctions for women and doctors making abortion legal on request up to 16 weeks. In New South Wales two court rulings liberalized the law. These were the Levine Ruling of 1971 and the Kirby ruling of 1994. Western Australia passed a law on 29 May 1998 which allowed abortion on request until 20 weeks, the only condition being that a woman must undergo counselling by a medical practitioner other than the one performing the operation.

Many have regarded Queensland as the most conservative of the states. For example in 1977 it banned street assemblies. After an anti-abortion group had failed in an attempt to impose the existing law on a clinic in Brisbane an effort was made to introduce a very conservative law. It would allow abortion only for rape or incest after police investigations but not, for example, the contraction of rubella in the early stages of pregnancy. A doctor who advised a woman to go to New South Wales for an abortion would be regarded as frustrating the objects of the act (Section 19) and could be struck off the medical register. The Bill was opposed by 3,000 women who defied the street assembly ban and was also opposed by the Australian Medical Association. In the event 19 members of the Government crossed the floor to oppose the bill and secure its defeat (Francome 1984, p. 152). In 2002 the Australian Capital Territory removed abortion from its penal code (Katzive 2007). In practice, first-trimester abortion is available on request everywhere in Australia.

In 2012, mifepristone was approved for terminating pregnancies after many years of attempts by women's groups to make medication abortion available. The application was made by MSI, a nonprofit service provider, rather than a pharmaceutical company, presumably because the potential profits would not justify the cost of the application. (*NPS Medicinewise* (2012) 'Mifepristone-misoprostol TGA listed', NPS Direct).

There is no abortion reporting requirement except in South Australia, so the number of abortions must be estimated from medical insurance reimbursements and hospital records. One set of estimates shows the number of abortions in Australia declining from 77,060 in 2001 to 62,820 in 2010. During this time the number of live births had increased from 246,000 to 298,000. Consequently, the percentage of pregnancies ending in abortion declined from 23.9 per cent to 17.4 per cent.

New Zealand

The population was estimated at 4.4 million in 2013 and life expectancy at birth was 80.8 years. Its religion is 44 per cent Protestant, 13 per cent Catholic. A third (32 per cent) had no religion and an additional one in ten had an unspecified religion. In 2011 the average woman had 2.1 children. The capital city is Wellington with a population of 391,000 (2009), the biggest city is Auckland with a population of 1.4 million (CIA 2013, p. 525).

As in Australia the abortion law in New Zealand was modelled on the British 1861 Offences Against the Person Act. It was known that historically illegal abortions occurred and also that doctors could carry out some abortions legally to protect the woman's physical or mental health. A committee of enquiry was set up under D.G. McMilland and this reported in 1936 that one in five pregnancies ended in an abortion. They were very often unsafe at this time and in 1934 at least 42 women died. The introduction of antibiotics in the 1940s made infection less likely and so probably increased the number. The British 1967 Abortion Act stirred debate in New Zealand as did the legalization in South Australia in 1969. This legislation was particularly important because in meant that New Zealand women who could afford to travel could have a safe operation (Francome 1984, p. 152).

A major development was the setting up of the Auckland Medical Aid Centre in May 1974. This aimed to provide cheap abortions, and though reports said 80 per cent of GPs had referred patients to it there were several attempts to close it (*Guardian* 24 October 1978). Opposition to a liberal abortion act was relatively strong, and the Society for the Protection of the Unborn Child (SPUC) was formed in 1970. By May 1975, SPUC was able to organize an 8,000 strong march on Parliament. A Royal Commission on abortion was set up in 1975 as a result of the furore provoked by the setting up of the Auckland Centre. It reported in 1977 and had a strong anti-abortion leaning. It led to the 'Contraception, Sterilization and Abortion Act later in the year. The Auckland Centre immediately closed, and although a limited number of abortion services remained availably, the Sisters Overseas Service (SOS) arranged for women to fly to Australia once more. The need for this service ended when the Auckland Centre re-opened, and by 1980 the abortion rates were back to the 1976 level (Francome 1984, p. 154).

The anti-abortion group SPUC split in 1983. The Christchurch group were more extreme and copied the absolutists in the US. In fact in the mid-eighties the Chicago-based anti-abortion activist Joseph Scheidler visited New Zealand and prompted the formation of self-styled 'pro-life action groups' in Wellington and Christchurch. However, things have calmed down in recent years.

The 1977 act permits abortions to protect the woman's mental and physical health and in cases of rape and foetal impairment. In practice, abortion is generally available on request. The Abortion Law Reform Association of New Zealand (ALRANZ) wants abortion to be wholly decriminalized and a bill to do this was proposed in 2010 and may return. As in Australia there has been a fall in the number of abortions. The number of abortions and the abortion rate rose steadily to a peak in 2003, when they were 18,511 and 20.8 per 1,000, respectively, and have since fallen to 14,745 and 16.1 in 2012. In that year, 19.3 per cent of pregnancies ended in abortion (Statistics New Zealand (2013) 'Abortion Statistics: Year ended December 2012; http://www.stats.govt.nz/browse_for_stats/health/abortion/AbortionStatistics_HOTPYeDec12.aspx), a rate that is slightly higher than Australia but is similar to the figure estimated for 1936 (Johnston 2013q).

Papua New Guinea

The population of Papua New Guinea was estimated to be 6.4 million in 2013 and its life expectancy from birth was 66.7 years. It gained its independence from Australia in September 1975. Seven out of ten (69 per cent) of the population are Protestant and 27 per cent Catholic (2000 census, CIA 2014, p. 564) The country is the world's second biggest island and because of the fact its population is disparate and a total of 850 languages are spoken. In 2013 the average woman had 3.3 children which is a reduction of 0.6 from 2005. Its capital is Port Moresby with a population of 314,000 (2009 estimate).

As there are many different cultures within the country there are a variety of patterns of relationships. However, overall researchers claim that the average age of first intercourse for both sexes is around 15 or 16 years. Reports indicate some strange beliefs which can affect the number of unwanted pregnancies. For example, many people believe pregnancy will not occur until couples have sex at least six times. Local observers suggest this leads to people changing their partners frequently in order to avoid pregnancy (Oliver-Miller 2004).

The high maternal mortality rate is in part due to the lack of care in rural areas. So while 88 per cent of urban women have a birth attendant it is only the case for 48 per cent of rural women. Lack of medical care is also likely to be a factor in that one in 25 women who reached the age of 12 would eventually die of maternal factors. The figure for urban areas was one in 35 (World Bank 2013a).

In 2006 both MSI and Pathfinder International started providing contraceptive services. MSI developed an outreach team which set off on a Monday morning and returned at the end of the week. It provided a mobile clinic and presentations for sometimes over a hundred people at a time. Contraceptives are provided at a heavily subsidized price. In 2006–2007, 32 per cent of women were using a contraceptive method.

Abortion is illegal but the number seems to have been increasing. Consequently one observer comments 'It is not unusual to hear about young girls and older women inducing abortions'. However, these often lead to serious infections and even the death of the woman. The abortions are usually carried out by herbs, inserting things like sticks into the vagina or even tying a rope around the abdomen. In 2013 a conference sponsored by the UN expressed concern at the high levels of unsafe abortions. Lisa Vallely, head of maternal and child health commented: 'No one knows the actual numbers but it is clear that the number of school age girls (having an unsafe abortion) is unacceptably high' (IRIN 2013).

Timor Leste

The country declared itself independent from Portugal in 1975 but was then occupied by Indonesia. In 2002 it became fully recognized as an independent state. Since that time it has had some troubles, including an attempted attack on the President and Prime Minister in 2008. The ringleader of the rebels was killed in the incident and there has been a period of stability. Life expectancy from birth was 67.1 in 2013 which is a remarkable increase from 42.5 years in 1990. The infant mortality rate of 40.1 is a reduction from 166 in 1990. The country is 98 per cent Catholic (2005) and its capital city is Dili with a population of 166,000 (2009). In 2011 the average woman had 3.1 children.

A local informant said she became involved in helping provide reproductive health services in the country. 'I felt compelled to work in reproductive health so as to help alleviate poverty and infant and maternal mortality in Timor Leste'. Another commented 'During the process of separation the health service was much damaged and reproductive health was not a great priority' (Francome and Vekemans 2004, p. 118).

The cost of condoms is high relative to local income; however, in 2007 the Ministry of Health and UNFPA began providing free condoms in community health centres. Marie Stopes International went to the country in 2006 and began its outreach programme in April 2007 Abortion is illegal in the country except to save the life of the woman. Consequently, many of the abortions are carried out clandestinely. Our respondent commented: 'Traditional methods of abortion are used but they are shrouded in secrecy. Illegal abortion frequently causes a need for post abortion care'.

A report in 2009 said there was pressure for more lenient abortion laws from a group called Fokupers (Communication Forum for Women from the East), a local organization supported by the Alola Foundation. A Fokupers spokeswoman Maria Barreto told attendees at a conference:

> Abortion is one of the options that is appropriate when the mothers are victims of sexual violence. We are working to protect women. We should understand that we should give options to mothers based on their circumstances.

She continued to say that incest was common in remote areas where parents and children often slept in the same room. The conference called for relatively minor change in the law, but the Catholic Church is opposed to any relaxation of the statute. The Catholic Church did however, support mothers' spacing their children, although not by using modern contraceptive methods (IRIN Asia 2013). One nun was quoted as saying,'the Pope says 'No' so we must follow what he says. If I were free I would do it' (Belton et al. 2009).

Vanuatu (Formerly New Hebrides)

The population consists of 12 major and 60 smaller islands in the Pacific Ocean. Their population was estimated at 261,565 in 2013, and the life expectancy at birth was 72.4 years. Seven out of ten (69.4 per cent) residents are Protestant, 13 per cent Catholic and eight per cent subscribe to indigenous beliefs. In the year 2003 the birth rate was 26 per 1,000; this fell to 21 in 2011. In 1970 the country had a family size of 6.5 children per woman. By 2005 the average woman had only 3.9 children and in 2013 it was down to 3.5, a remarkable reduction (though the World Bank gives a higher figure). Its capital is Port Vila (CIA 2013, p. 784).

Family Planning was part of the country's programme on its independence in 1980. The World Bank gave figures that the percentage of women using contraception was 38 per cent of those aged 15–49 in 1995 but then fell to 28 per cent in 1999 before rising again to 38 per cent in 2007 (World Bank 2011). A conference of Pacific groups occurred in 2012 and Dr Elisa Kennedy of Melbourne said that Vanuatu needed $6.2 million to improve contraceptive funding. In the following year Kennedy and colleagues published an article making the case for investing in family planning in the Pacific. They calculated that meeting family planning needs by 2020 would increase the prevalence of modern contraception by 2025 in Vanuatu from 36.8 per cent to 65.5. It would also lead to a fertility decline from 4.1 births per woman down to 2.2 (Kennedy 2013). The abortion law is restrictive, allowing abortion to protect the physical health of the pregnant woman but not for rape, incest or foetal problems. In 2005, the death of three young babies, possibly unnecessarily, led to concerns that many women were not getting the support they needed. Mrs Merilyn Tahi of the Women's Crisis Centre called upon the government to revise the abortion law. She pointed out that many women went abroad for their operations and of course it could only be the richer women who had the resources to do so (Radio Vanuatu 11 May).

The lack of adequate family planning resources led the leaders of the country's services to welcome the extra supplies pledged in the 2012 London Conference. Emily Bevu of Vanuatu FHA said that a lack of contraceptives was putting women's lives at risk and that dire consequences could follow as unwanted pregnancies led to them seeking illegal abortions.

Conclusion

The area has undergone rapid change. In the twentieth century Margaret Mead's famous book *Coming of Age in Samoa* was a study of a primitive people who had a relaxed attitude towards sex from which she felt Americans could learn. When towards the end of the twentieth century the Samoans beat the Welsh at rugby football, we realized that the country had come into the modern world in a short time. There is still poverty and illiteracy amongst the poor countries of the area. However, the closeness of the poorer countries to Australia and New Zealand raises their awareness of the wealth towards which they might aspire, as well as allowing them to observe the advantages of developed societies. So we may expect rapid changes to continue in the area.

Chapter 7
North America

'A full generation of Canadians has lived without a law and we are better off for it'.
(Joyce Arthur 2013)

The birthrate for this region has remained largely remained constant at 2.0 children per woman. It did drop slightly to 1.9 children in 1990–95, but otherwise has been remarkably stable.

Canada

In 2013 the population was 34.6 million people and its fertility rate was 1.6 children per woman, which was a slight increase from seven years earlier. The majority of the Canadian population identifies as either Roman Catholic (43 per cent), Protestant (28 per cent), other (12 per cent), or Muslim (2 per cent), while 16 per cent claim no religious affiliation (2001 census). Canada's population is concentrated in the southern part of the country with over 80 per cent living in urban areas (CIA 2014, p. 133).

From 1869 onward, abortion providers faced life imprisonment while any woman inducing her own abortion could be sentenced to seven years incarceration (Childbirth by Choice Trust 1998). In 1892 the government was influenced by the passage of restrictive US laws on birth control and prohibited the sale, advertisement and dissemination of contraceptives and abortifacients (McLaren and McLaren 1997). From 1926–1947, 4,000–6,000 women died of unsafe abortions because the illegality of the operation forced women to self-abort or to seek out clandestine, medical or non-medical personnel (Arthur 2013). While most women survived, many died from subsequent infections. By the 1960s, abortion was a leading case of maternal death in some provinces. In a case in 1964 a mother of three children died of an illegal abortion and at the inquest the jury said that the law should be revised. In 1969, the Government under the leadership of Pierre Trudeau, later to become Prime Minister, reformed the criminal code. It decriminalized contraception and homosexuality and legalized abortion where continuation of the pregnancy 'would or would be likely to' endanger the life or health of the pregnant woman. Trudeau commented 'The state has no business in the bedrooms of the nation' (Arthur 2013).

Although this law made legal abortion more available, the process of getting an abortion under the law was very bureaucratic. The procedure had to take place in a hospital and be approved by a Therapeutic Basis Abortion Committee composed of three to five physicians. The committee would determine if an abortion were necessary on a case by case basis. Only about a third of hospitals established these committees, and those that did were located primarily in urban centres. There were also weaknesses in the system as doctors were not always willing to serve in the abortion process and furthermore the definition of 'health' varied tremendously. Some committees rarely approved an abortion, while others routinely allowed them. Although the law was somewhat restrictive, the number of recorded abortions increased from 11,000 in 1970 to 43,000 in 1973 (Francome 1984, p. 154).

The opposition of pro-choice feminists, physicians and activists to the restrictions of the 1969 law coalesced around Dr Henry Morgentaler, a Montreal physician. Morgentaler repeatedly broke the law by terminating pregnancies in abortion clinics he established in Montreal, Toronto and Winnipeg.

The law might have continued with a gradual liberalization had it not been for the prosecution of Dr Morgentaler in Quebec, a province where it was very difficult to obtain a legal abortion. A first prosecution in 1970 came to nothing. Morgentaler carried out over 6,000 abortions between 1969 and 1973 outside of a hospital and without going through the legality of the medical committee. In August of that year a police raid led to him being prosecuted again. Morgentaler relied on the 'Good Samaritan provision of the Criminal Code, which protects a person carrying out surgery for another's benefit if it is reasonable to perform the operation having regard to the state of health of the person at the time the operation is performed and to all the circumstances of the case' (Francome 1984, p. 154). He was acquitted by the jury but in a clear breach of common law rights the Quebec Court of Appeal ordered a conviction. This was upheld by the Canadian Supreme Court and in March 1975 Morgentaler went to prison to serve ten months of an 18-month sentence. This he continued to serve even after the government in Ottawa undertook in July 1975 to change the law to prevent any further appeal court ordering convictions after a jury trial. When I met Morgentaler in Washington DC in 1978 he told me he had been responsible for a change in the law called the 'Morgentaler Amendment'. As he sat in prison after his 'not guilty' verdict, at least he could take comfort from the fact that it would not happen to anyone else. In 1975 Morgentaler was prosecuted again and for the third time the jury refused to convict him. This time the Quebec Court of Appeal upheld his acquittal. The Province of Quebec decided the law was unenforceable and established a network of local medical clinics where abortions were performed in contravention of the national law.

Dr Morgentaler then opened clinics in other provinces. When he was prosecuted in Ontario, the case went to the Supreme Court under the title *R* v *Morgentaler*. In a landmark decision in 1988, the Court declared the entire abortion law to violate Canada's Charter of Rights and Freedoms, which was enacted in 1982. Thus Canada is one of the few countries with no reference to abortion in its criminal law. In its decision the Court commented:

> The decision whether or not to terminate a pregnancy is essentially a moral decision and in a free and democratic society, the conscience of the individual must be paramount to that of the state.

On 28 January 2013 it was the 25th anniversary of decriminalization. Joyce Arthur, the executive director of the Abortion Rights Coalition of Canada commented: 'A full generation of Canadians has lived without a law and we are better off for it'. She continued to say that the Canadian Medical Association had successfully managed abortion like all other medical procedures with a strong code of ethics and further maintained that criminal laws are inappropriate in the medical area as they interfere with good health. She continued to say that even though there are no restrictions, after 20 weeks abortions are performed only for severe foetal abnormality or for compelling maternal health reasons.

Data reveals that in 2003 103,768 legal abortions were performed but the number had declined to 92,524 in 2011 (Statistics Canada 2007a and Canadian Institute for Health Information http://www.cihi.ca/cihi-ext-portal/pdf/internet/ta_11_alldatatables20130221_en, accessed 21 June 2014). Although reporting is incomplete in some provinces, it is clear that abortion numbers and rates have declined in recent years.

Since 1988 abortion is not only legal, but is also fully funded as a medically necessary service under the Canada Health Act. This requires that medically necessary services be accessible, portable, universal, comprehensive and publicly administered. Therefore, any restrictions on access to abortions technically violates the terms of the Act.

United States

Population was estimated at 317 million in 2013 and life expectancy was 78.6 years. The infant mortality rate was 5.9 per 1,000 births and maternal mortality rate was 21 per 100,000 live births. Its religion is 55 per cent Protestant and 24 per cent Catholic, two per cent Jewish and 19 per cent none or unaffiliated. Less than one per cent is either Muslim or Buddhist. In the year 2013 the birth rate was 13 per 1,000 and the death rate 8 per 1,000. This gives a rate of natural increase of 0.5 per cent. The fertility rate, 1.88 children per woman in 2012, has fallen steadily since the world financial crisis began in 2007, when it was 2.12. The country consists of fifty states, the capital district (District of Columbia), Puerto Rico, and some minor territories.

The individual states made abortion illegal in the nineteenth century, primarily to protect women from untrained abortionists. Nevertheless, there were a high number of illegal operations, which led to a *New York Times* campaign against abortion in the 1870s (Francome 1984, p. 47). Dissemination of information about birth control was also made illegal in 1873.

The first person to systematically argue for legalization of abortion was William Robinson, the editor of the journal *Critic and Guide* in 1913. He called for its decriminalization in the early stages of pregnancy, but disagreed with a German Professor Kocks who wanted it legalized for the duration of the pregnancy

(Francome 1984, p. 75). Robinson felt that abortion should only be used sparingly and this led him to be critical of some of the young people of his day.

> I do dislike a certain type of modern young woman who indulges promiscuously, uses contraception rather reluctantly, preferring repeat abortions which she regards as lightly as downing a cocktail or a glass of whisky. (Francome and Vekemans 2007, p. 133)

Robinson called for the legalization of abortion in at least two books and was supported in his wish to reform the laws by a woman's group which formed the Association for the Reform of the Abortion Laws in 1932 (Taussig 1936, p. 426). This group aimed to broaden grounds to include cases of rape, seduction, infirmity, likely handicap, destitution and divorce. However, such calls were unsuccessful in a society when the doctor's main medical association did not accept contraception until 1937 (Francome 1984, p. 76). So at the outbreak of the Second World War, abortion was illegal in every state but there were wide variations in penalties and provisions were not uniform. In six states there were no legal exemptions. In thirty-nine states abortion was legal to save the life of the woman and in a further three states and the District of Columbia abortion was also allowed for the health of the woman. In Mississippi alone the operation was legal at the discretion of the medical practitioner (Birkett, 1939, p. 165).

Changing the Law

In the post-war years the early pressure was for the abortion law to be extended but not as far as to allow abortion on request. In December 1959 the American Law Institute circulated a model bill that would legalize abortion if continuation of the pregnancy would 'gravely impair the physical or mental health of the mother,' for rape or incest, and for foetal abnormality. In the 1960s, a movement to liberalize abortion laws was prompted in part by a rubella epidemic that resulted in some 15,000 infants born with birth defects. When nine respected doctors in California were threatened with the loss of their licenses for providing abortions to rubella patients, physicians and prominent citizens nationally came to their defence. A happily married mother of four who was forced to fly to Sweden for an abortion after taking thalidomide also received widespread sympathetic publicity. In 1967 the American Medical Association decided to support the American Law Institute model bill.

The first state to expand the grounds for abortion was Colorado in 1967, followed by California and North Carolina. In 1968 Georgia and Maryland liberalized their laws and in 1969 so did Arkansas, Kansas, Delaware, Oregon and New Mexico. By this time of course rich women could obtain legal abortions in Britain or illegal but safe abortions in Puerto Rico. The first state to pass a law allowing abortion on request was Hawaii in 1970, however, this law required the woman to be a resident of the state. Similar laws were passed in Alaska and Washington.

It was the dramatic legalization of abortion on request up to 24 weeks in New York State that made abortion available to practically all women in the eastern half of the country who had the resources to travel and pay for the procedure. Governor Rockefeller and many state legislators favoured an expansion of the grounds for abortion, but Catholic groups and other abortion opponents amended the proposal to allow abortion without restriction as to reason in the belief that this would kill the bill. Surprisingly, the bill passed the State Senate and the vote was tied in the state assembly. At the last minute, under the influence of his wife and daughters, one assemblyman raised his hand and changed his vote in favour of the bill. He said at the time that this vote would cost him his seat in the assembly, and this in fact happened at the next election. Hundreds of thousands of women came from all over the country for services in New York in 1971 and 1972.

In 1972 the Massachusetts law banning birth control for single people was overthrown by the Supreme Court on the grounds of privacy. This was one of the factors which paved the way for the Supreme Court decision of 22 January 1973, which made all abortion laws in the US unconstitutional. The decision – *Roe v. Wade* – divided pregnancy into trimesters. In the first abortion was legal on the grounds of privacy and the decision left to the woman and her attending physician. After this time, however, the interests of the state in promoting the health of the woman became of increased importance and so states could regulate abortion procedures in ways that were reasonably related to maternal health. Once viability had been reached the states could proscribe abortion in pursuit of its interest in the potential human life except when it was necessary to preserve the life or health of the woman (Osofsky and Osofsky, 1973).

US After the 1973 Supreme Court Decision

The legal ruling meant that even states most opposed to liberal laws were prevented from keeping their legislation. Even the New York law which allowed abortion until 24 weeks was unconstitutional. The strength of feeling against the decision can be gauged by the fact that the legislature in the Mormon stronghold of Utah condemned the decision by 66 votes to 1.

During the 1970s and 1980s, the Supreme Court found many restrictions enacted by states were unconstitutional under *Roe v. Wade*. Then in 1992, in the case of *Planned Parenthood of Southeastern Pennsylvania v. Casey*, the Supreme Court relaxed the standards that restrictions have to meet in order to be constitutional. In that case, it held that although women still have the right to terminate a pregnancy as established by *Roe v. Wade*, restrictions are permissible as long as they do not constitute an 'undue burden' on women, that is, they do not have the purpose or effect of placing a substantial obstacle in the path of a woman seeking an abortion. We can consider some areas where restrictions have been attempted.

Medicaid Coverage Unavailable for Abortion Services

In 1977, Congress eliminated coverage of most abortions under the national health insurance plan for poor families. The Supreme Court held that the government has no constitutional responsibility to provide funds for medically necessary abortions. Currently the 'Hyde Amendment' prohibits federal payment for abortions other than those for pregnancies caused by rape, incest or those necessary to save the woman's life. Nevertheless, some states continue to pay for most medically necessary abortions under their Medicaid programs without the benefit of federal funding.

Parental Notification or Consent for Minors

In *Bellotti v Baird*, 1979, and other decisions, the Supreme Court held that unemancipated minors could be required to notify one or both parents or obtain their consent before obtaining an abortion, provided that an alternative is available that prevent parents from having an absolute ability to block the abortion. In most cases, the alternative is access to a judge, who must grant the abortion request if the minor is mature enough to make an informed decision or if the abortion is in the minor's best interest. As of 2014, 21 states require that minors obtain the consent of one or both parents, 12 that one or both parents be notified, and 5 require both parental consent and notification. Eight states require the parental consent documentation to be notarized. All of these states provide for a judicial bypass and seven also have provision for notice or consent of another adult relative (Guttmacher Institute 2014). In some states the judicial bypass procedure works smoothly, often with the help of volunteer lawyers, while in others bypasses are almost never granted.

Although the asserted purpose of these laws is to encourage minors to consult their parents before having an abortion, there is little evidence that this has been accomplished where judicial bypass is available. One study compared the proportion of minors who consulted parents on Minnesota, where a requirement was in effect, with Wisconsin, where there was no requirement. It found little difference in the proportion of minors whose parents knew about their abortions. In the absence of any law, about 60 per cent of minors say one or both parents are aware that they are having abortions. The proportion is higher among younger teenagers, reaching as high as 90 per cent of those under age 14 (Henshaw and Kost 1992). One immediate effect of the laws, however, is that minors travel to neighbouring states to avoid parental involvement requirements or to states with less stringent requirements. A study of the effect of a Massachusetts parental consent law found that the number of Massachusetts minors having abortions in Rhode Island, New Hampshire, and other states rose significantly but there was little change in the total number of minors having abortions or births (Cartoof and Klerman 1986).

Similarly, studies in Mississippi and Missouri found increases in the number of minors obtaining abortion services in other states (Henshaw 1995). Another possible effect of parental involvement laws is that minors would continue more of their pregnancies, either because they consulted parents who favoured childbirth or because they delayed dealing with the pregnancy to the point where abortion was no longer possible. Studies in Massachusetts and Mississippi found little increase in the birth rates of minors, suggesting that any such effect would be minor (Cartoof and Klerman 1986, Henshaw 1995) One study that was able to take age into account found that among women who conceived at age 17, a larger proportion gave birth after a parental notice law went into effect in Texas (Joyce et al. 2006). Overall, however, the change was small. Another effect of the laws is to delay the minors who have abortions despite the requirements. Statistics from Minnesota and Mississippi show that parental involvement laws increase the proportion of minors whose abortions are beyond 12 weeks by about one-fifth (Rogers et al. 2001, Henshaw 1995). Delay could be caused by reluctance of the minors to go to court or involve their parents, the wait to see a judge, or the time needed to arrange for travel to other states. A study in Texas also found that women who were nearly 18 years old delayed their abortion until their 18th birthday. This resulted in an elevated number of later abortions among women exactly 18 years old (Joyce et al. 2006). Some proponents of parental involvement requirements believe that they prevent teenage pregnancy, either by reducing sexual activity or by causing minors to use contraception more conscientiously. Opponents of parental involvement laws have argued that they harm minors in some cases, especially where there is parental abuse or family conflict. No systematic research has been able to examine this question. A survey of minors having abortions in states without parental involvement requirements found that conflict occurred when parents found out about the abortion without being told by the pregnant girl. Severe consequences resulted in a small proportion of these cases. These included the minor suffering physical violence and being forced to leave home. In sum, parental involvement laws clearly cause delay and out-of-state travel, and they result in an unknown level of family conflict that is harmful to the women. In a few cases, they may result in families causing minors to continue unwanted pregnancies. The benefits of increased parental support and pregnancy prevention are difficult to measure.

State-mandated Counselling and Waiting Periods

An increasing number of states, 35 as of 2014, require that women receive counselling before an abortion is performed. Twenty-seven detail the specific information the woman must be given. This communication frequently includes the risks of abortion and childbirth, a description of foetal development, the assistance available to women for prenatal care, childbirth, and infant care, and a list of agencies that provide information or services designed to help women carry their pregnancies to term. A few states require women to be told that having an abortion may increase the risk of breast cancer. This is despite the fact that medical authorities are in agreement that no such relationship exists. Twelve states require that women be told that a foetus at 20 weeks or more may feel pain and be offered anaesthesia for the foetus, and eight require that women be told of possible negative psychological impacts of abortion but not of positive consequences. A majority of the states require that mandated counselling must take place a specified number of hours, usually 24, before the abortion can be performed. Eleven states require that the information be delivered in person, which means that in most cases the woman must make two trips to the abortion facility. A number of states require the woman to be offered the opportunity to see the ultrasound of her embryo or foetus (Guttmacher Institute, 2014).

The Supreme Court held in 1983 in *City of Akron v. Akron Center* for Reproductive Health that state-directed counselling and waiting period requirements are unconstitutional and reaffirmed this decision with respect to counselling in 1986 in *Thornburgh v. American College of Obstetricians and Gynecologists*, Pennsylvania Section. Nevertheless, it overruled these decisions in Casey in 1992, when it found that required counselling and waiting periods did not violate the new 'undue burden' criterion. Although proponents of these requirements say they are needed to help women make informed decisions, the implicit purpose is to discourage abortion. Evidence for this is that no similar requirements apply to women seeking prenatal care, though the decision to continue a pregnancy carries more risk and responsibility than the decision to terminate a pregnancy. Abortion providers have found that the required counselling and waiting periods have little effect on women's abortion decisions, although they object in principle to the assumption that women need special constraints when making important decisions and that the state can override the judgment of medical professionals about the information needed by their patients. It is not clear whether the required counselling succeeds in evoking guilt in women having abortions. The two-trip requirement, however, may be a significant burden and prevent some women from obtaining desired abortion services. A study of abortion statistics from Mississippi and neighbouring states found that approximately 11 per cent of the women who would have had abortions were prevented from doing so by a two-trip requirement. In addition, many women went to other states to avoid the requirement, and abortions were delayed on average (Joyce et al. 2006) In summary, the counselling and waiting period requirements appear to serve little purpose except to act as a barrier to services, to increase costs, and possibly to further stigmatize abortion.

Clinic Licensing and Other Restrictions on Abortion Facilities

In the 1960s, abortion was considered a dangerous procedure that should be performed in hospitals. After the law was liberalized in New York in 1970, hospitals were unable to meet the demand, so clinics were established that used a simpler and safer procedure – vacuum aspiration. Studies in the 1970s demonstrated that first and early second-trimester abortions in non-hospital clinics are as safe as those performed in hospitals. Today only four per cent of abortions take place in hospital inpatient or outpatient departments. In the Akron and other decisions the Supreme Court held that states could not require that all second-trimester abortions be performed in hospitals. However, laws requiring that clinics be licensed and meet strict standards for the facility and staff have generally not been found to be unconstitutional. Despite the excellent safety record of abortion clinics, a number of states have recently imposed burdensome licensing requirements. In many cases, clinics must meet the standards of ambulatory surgical centres, which often approach the standards of hospitals. For example, the standards specify the amount of air flow, the size of corridors, the number and location of toilets and dressing areas for staff, and the like. These standards apply to abortions performed by the administration of medications as well as surgical abortions. Given the safety of abortion, it is unlikely that such measures improve the safety of abortions or that they prevent deaths or complications.

A new requirement imposed by several states is that each physician performing abortions must have admitting privileges at a local hospital. This provision has forced the closing of many clinics because of the difficulties doctors face in obtaining hospital privilege. In Mississippi, for example, no physician is willing to offer abortion services, so the one clinic's physician flies in from a distant state, and hospitals rarely grant privileges to a physician who does not live in the area. Some cities have no hospitals who will grant privileges to an abortion provider, and some physicians are ineligible because they do not admit the required number of patients, usually at least ten a year. No physician should need to admit more than one or two patients a year for abortion complications. A related requirement in nine states is that abortion providers have a transfer agreement with a hospital for emergency cases. This requirement is unnecessary because hospitals are required to accept all emergency cases.

Protection of Access to Clinic Entrances

In the mid-1980s, anti-abortion protests became increasingly violent and destructive. Bombings, arson, vandalism, blockades and violent protests were relatively common. In 1994, the federal government enacted the Freedom of Access to Clinic Entrances Act, which prohibits the use of force or physical obstruction to interfere with someone entering a reproductive health care facility. This act, together with other factors such as the increasing political success of anti-abortion forces, is credited with a reduction in clinic violence. In addition to the federal law, some 15 states and the District of Columbia prohibit certain anti-abortion activities directed at abortion providers such as blocking of clinic entrances and intimidating staff. Several places have protected "bubble zones", regions of a specified number of feet around a person within a certain distance of a clinic that cannot be entered by a protester without the person's consent.

Other Abortion-related Policies

Other issues affect abortion providers and access to abortion services. Nine states prohibit private health insurance from covering abortion services except in a rider with an additional charge, and 25 others restrict abortion coverage in plans that are offered under the new national health insurance program. A majority of states require that abortions be performed by physicians even though studies have shown that first-trimester vacuum aspirations can be performed safely by mid-level practitioners (midwives, physician assistants, and nurse clinicians). A few states, most recently California, have mid-level practitioners performing abortions In some states abortion services may not be performed in any public facilities, including state medical school hospitals. Requirements about the disposal of foetal remains increase providers' costs in some states. Three states have policies in effect that make it virtually impossible to provide first-trimester medication abortions (that is, by mifepristone). Several states prohibit abortions past 20 weeks or after a foetal heartbeat can be detected. The constitutionality of these restrictions is being tested.

Policy Trends

Changes in the structure of the Supreme Court may result in relaxation of the limits on the extent to which abortion can be restricted. On most issues, the court is sharply divided into four very conservative justices who would probably reverse *Roe v. Wade*, four more liberal justices, and one moderately conservative justice who provided the deciding vote in many cases. While it is possible that *Roe v. Wade* could be reversed, the predominant thinking is that the Court could permit more severe restrictions without entirely overruling *Roe v. Wade*. However, it is difficult to predict how the swing justice will decide abortion issues.

The Practice of Legal Abortion

The number of abortions peaked at 1.6 million a year in 1990 and has since fallen to 1.1 million by 2011 according to the Guttmacher Institute. Abortion rates are relatively high in large metropolitan areas and low in small towns and rural areas. This may be in part because of greater availability of abortion services in metropolitan areas and the barrier posed by long distances in some parts of the country. Abortion rates are high among black women (50 per 1,000) and Hispanic women (22) in comparison with non-Hispanic white women (10). (National Center for Health Statistics (2013) *Data Brief Number 136*) Other groups with especially high abortion rates are women aged 18–24, never-married women, cohabiting women, and those with low income and those eligible for Medicaid health insurance (Jones, Darroch and Henshaw (2002).

The abortion rate has been falling slowly in recent years, mainly because of a reduction among teenagers and a decrease in the proportion of unintended pregnancies ending in abortion. Going against the overall trend are increasing unintended pregnancy and abortion rates among women whose income is below 200 per cent of the federal poverty standard and among cohabiting women (Finer and Henshaw 2006). Prenatal screening followed by abortion when necessary has allowed couples to avoid the birth of children with congenital abnormalities. The result is a marked decrease in the number of such births. The number of children born in 2001 with Down's Syndrome was 3,654, about half the number that would be expected in the absence of screening (Egan et al. 2004). About half of women choose to continue pregnancies when abnormalities are identified. However, for some of those who end such pregnancies, the birth of a disabled child would be devastating psychologically, socially and economically.

A factor in recent years is the increasing use of long-acting reversible contraception, especially the IUD (intra-uterine device) and implant. More clinicians are emphasizing the use-effectiveness of these methods because no effort is required of the user. With the recent health insurance reform that provides contraceptive coverage for more women, the cost barriers should disappear and the rate of unintended pregnancy should decline. The abortion rate may decline even more as service availability declines due to the closing of clinics that cannot meet the new requirements.

Appendix

Challenging Abortion Restrictions

Many challenges to state abortion restrictions have been brought in federal courts over the years and have often been successful in having restrictions declared unconstitutional and unenforceable. Recently enacted requirements that physicians who perform abortions have admitting privileges at local hospitals have forced the closing of almost half of the abortion facilities in Texas and clinics in other states. This spring (2014), lawyers for the American Civil Liberties Union (ACLU) and Planned Parenthood asked me to testify as an expert witness in federal lawsuits against similar laws in two states, Alabama and Wisconsin.

The legal argument is two-fold: that the requirement does little or nothing to improve patient safety, and that forcing women to travel longer distances because clinics have been closed constitutes an "undue burden" on abortion rights. In addition, the lawyers need to show that it would be difficult or impossible for the physicians to obtain local hospital privileges.

The heart of my testimony was that, if the restrictions forced the closing of clinics, some of the women who would have been served by those clinics would have to travel between 60 and 100 miles farther for abortion care and that a substantial proportion of those women would be unable to go the extra distance. The state attorneys argued that many women already travel long distances for abortions and other health care, and that such travel is normal for them. What they overlook are the many women who fail to make the trip and therefore do not appear in any statistics.

My first task was to review the literature for research measuring the impact of distance. There are many studies that have found a strong correlation between the availability of local abortion services and the local abortion rate, but economists would argue that the abortion clinics might have been established in places with the greatest demand rather than the demand being increased by the presence of services. The ideal studies therefore show a change in the abortion rate in a location where facilities were started or closed. I chose five studies for the basis of my testimony, four of which have before-and-after data. The fifth, though cross-sectional, had enough statistical controls that I consider it to be credible. The lawyers asked me to be prepared to testify as to how many women would be prevented from obtaining abortions. Based on the studies, I judged that a distance of 100 miles would be an insurmountable barrier to at least 20 to 25 per cent of the women who would have had abortions.

Court proceedings can be a lengthy and gruelling process. I wrote an initial expert report describing my opinions and the studies on which they were based. Then an expert for the state wrote a report that attempted to discredit the studies on which I had based the report and that cited those with contrary findings. In the Alabama case, I responded with a rebuttal report answering his criticisms. He was disadvantaged because the evidence overwhelmingly supported my position, and most of the state expert's points were illogical or easily refuted.

Our strongest study was one documenting the result of a law in Texas that required all abortions past 15 weeks to be performed in hospitals or ambulatory surgical centres. When the law went into effect, none of the non-hospital facilities where most such abortions were performed were qualified as ambulatory surgical centres. The result was that Texas women needing abortions past 15 weeks had to go out of state, the average distance to the nearest out-of-state provider being 252 miles. The number of Texas women having abortions past 15 weeks, including the women who went to other states, then fell by 69 per cent. (The small number of abortions in Texas hospitals, which permit abortions only under special circumstances, did not increase.) The state's expert argued that clinics may have scheduled abortions to take place earlier (there was no change in earlier abortions except a slight increase at 15 weeks), and that the number of later abortions might have fallen even without the law (but there was no precedent for such a decline and no such decline in other US states at the time). The authors of this excellent study examined and ruled out every explanation for the decline other than the effect of the distance women would have to travel.

Before each trial, I was subject to a deposition in which the states' lawyers questioned me about my background and my planned testimony. The purpose of the depositions is to allow each side to know what to expect at trial, but the lawyers also attempt to make the witness make concessions and inconsistent statements. In my case, they spent considerable time looking for ways to show that I would be biased by asking my personal opinions, my motivations for studying the issue, and my associations with pro-choice organizations. For example, they had located the wording of an award I won from a pro-choice organization ten years ago and asked why I was given the award. Fortunately, the statement I wrote in connection with the award emphasized my research rather than activism. I was asked if I had ever testified in favour of a restriction on abortion. My answer was that no, I wasn't aware of restrictions that would improve patient safety and that I saw no reason that abortion services should be regulated differently from other similar health care. They also tried to use me to support their point that requiring hospital privileges is a legitimate health measure by quoting a question we used in a 1981 survey of abortion clinics. The depositions were focused surprisingly little on the research I cited, either because the states' lawyers had little confidence dealing with statistical studies or they weren't aware of possible weaknesses in the studies.

The ACLU lawyers were present at the depositions, but had very little power to block inappropriate or embarrassing questions. The depositions each took three to six hours, much longer than my trial testimony. A court reporter produced a verbatim transcript of everything said, which was sent to me to review and correct for any errors. Any mistake or concession in a deposition can be brought up at the trial to discredit your testimony or show bias. I was advised to respond slowly to all questions to give myself time to consider the answer and to frustrate the questioner. (I was not really able to do this. My impulse to respond immediately was uncontrollable.) It happened that little of what I said in the depositions came up in my trial cross-examinations.

Testimony at trial is also stressful. In the direct examination by my lawyers, I needed to be careful to describe the research clearly and accurately so that the judges, who generally have little background in statistics, will understand. My lawyers were good about reminding me if I neglected to make an important point. In preparation for the cross-examination, my lawyers grilled me with every difficult or embarrassing question they could think of. Fortunately, most of these questions didn't come up. The depositions gave us an idea of what the state lawyers would ask.

The federal judges seemed receptive to our case, and I am hopeful that their decisions will be favourable. In both cases, the judges granted temporary restraining orders to prevent the laws from taking effect until after the final decisions. More uncertain is what the appeals courts will decide, and then, of course, the Supreme Court, because they can define "undue burden" however they wish.

Chapter 8
Conclusions and Recommendations

> 'If the Catholic Church is genuine about wishing to reduce the number of abortions it should support the policies of those countries with low abortion rates. These are the countries of Europe with good contraceptive facilities who support the right to choose'.

In affluent countries we can distinguish four groups. In countries like Belgium, Holland, Germany and Switzerland there are good quality contraceptive and abortion services and low abortion rates. In some ways they may provide an example as to what can be achieved in other countries by a change of policy. Secondly there are those countries which, while being rich still have relatively high rates of unwanted pregnancy and clearly have the opportunity to contraception and reduce the demand for abortion. The UK is a good example in that when it introduced free contraception it did not include men. A change in policy with condoms being provided free through general practitioners as part of a men's health programme would not only reduce unwanted pregnancies but help reduce the incidence of sexually transmitted infections. A third group is the countries of Eastern Europe which have not had a tradition of contraception and therefore had much higher abortion rates than exist elsewhere. Finally, the fourth group are the four developed countries – Ireland, Poland, Malta and the Vatican – which do not allow legal abortion where women who do not want to continue a pregnancy have to travel abroad to obtain an abortion, or if poor risk local, unsafe abortions.

Amongst the poor countries there are important regional groupings. We have seen that in Latin America there are poor contraceptive services and many unsafe abortions. However, there are signs that things may be about to change, especially with legalization in Mexico City and the court decision in Colombia. In Africa the great amount of poverty, ethnic and national differences and very often a strong gender divide indicates the need for a great injection of resources and improvement of health not only in the area of childbirth, but through all the population. Asia benefits from the fact that the dominant religions are more supportive of family planning. However, the position of women is generally inferior and in need of improvement.

Pro-choice is Pro-Life

We who are in the pro-choice movement are pro-life in many ways. First of all the provision of safe legal abortion will save the lives of many thousands of mothers and enable them to care more adequately for their families. At the time a legal abortion is to be performed there is a great opportunity for educating women into the methods of modern contraception and wider health issues. This can help to reduce the number of deaths of children in infancy or in childhood. We are also in favour of women being able to use such things as artificial insemination by donor or *in vitro* fertilization to enable childless women to have a family. We saw in the introduction that decisions inspired by the Catholic Church in Poland have led to the closing of an *in vitro* fertilization facility in Warsaw.

There are those people who believe that it is possible to persuade young people to be sexually abstinent until they have finished their education and get married. They take the view that if this were to happen, there would be no need for abortion amongst single people. The few women who broke the norms could either keep the baby or give it up for adoption to a family who would give it good quality care. They also argue there would also be no need for abortion amongst the married for families would accept children as they came. However, the evidence of this book shows that there is not one society that in any way approaches this model.

There is also evidence that the US House of Representatives has been highly critical of US 'abstinence only' educational programmes. According to the Waxman Report, out of 13 curricula studied 11 contained scientific errors and distortions. Examples of such errors were that a boy could impregnate a girl by touching her genitals, that 10 per cent of women who undergo abortion become sterile, that 50 per cent of gay male teenagers are HIV positive that condoms fail to prevent HIV 31 per cent of the time and result in pregnancy 13 per cent of the time. The report suggested that youth who pledge abstinence are significantly less likely to have informed choices (Law and Policy 2005, p. 182).

Anti-Abortion Myths

The anti-abortionists have been misleading the population by promoting false propaganda or extreme viewpoints without public support. I will give some examples.

Anti-abortionists may say 'A woman should not be able to have an abortion for rape'. In the words of Dr and Mrs Willke 'Isn't it twisted logic that would kill an unborn baby for the crime of his father'. Similarly on 26 September 2006 the Pope said that 'abortion is never justifiable' (Westen 2008). However, to force women to maintain such pregnancies against their will is extending the initial crime and bringing further trauma. Furthermore, we have seen the evidence from the Congo which has shown that children born of rape often have extremely difficult lives though rejection. It is true that sometimes Protestant anti-abortion leaders take the view that abortion should be allowed for rape and we have seen the US 'Gag' rule allows abortion for this reason.

Some anti-abortionists say 'When a woman has been raped most of the trauma has already occurred.' To quote Willke and Willke again 'Will she be able to live comfortably with the memory that she killed her developing baby'. However, experience does not show this to be true. For example, when in 1938 Dr Aleck Bourne performed an abortion on a girl aged 14 who had been raped, she was forever grateful to him and 30 years later sent him a letter of thanks.

Anti-abortionists may oppose state funding for family planning. For example Robert G. Marshall, legislative counsel for the so-called U.S. Coalition for Life, stated in his testimony before Congress on the extension of the Health Services Act 1977 'We are opposed to the continued funding of the so-called family planning services and Population Research Act … both the IUD and one mode of action of the current pill are abortifacients'. However, scientific studies show that the IUD works primarily by preventing fertilization and oral contraceptives by blocking ovulation. In any case, we take the view that if poor do not have the right to control their own fertility they are denied an essential freedom. We can agree with the U.S. Supreme Court comments (22 January 1973):

> We recognize the right of the individual, married or single, to be free from the unwarranted governmental intrusion into matters so fundamentally affecting a person as the decision whether to bear or beget a child. That right necessarily included the right of a woman to decide whether or not to terminate a pregnancy.

Anti-abortionists may believe that the availability of birth control and abortion may lead to promiscuity. However, in Britain the evidence from Brook Advisory Service, which specializes in providing services to young people, shows that over 90 per cent of single people attending have already had intercourse.

Anti-abortionists may argue that the spreading of knowledge of birth control will not reduce unwanted pregnancies. For example on the fifth anniversary of the Supreme Court's decision legalizing abortion Bishop Joseph Bernadin said in *The New York Times* that he very much doubted whether,

> more and better contraceptive information and services will make major inroads in the number of teenage pregnancies … (for) it will motivate them to precocious sexual activity but by no means the practice of contraception. In which case the 'solution' will merely have made the problem worse.

However, we have seen many countries have improved contraceptive usage and reduced the number of unwanted pregnancies. For example in England and Wales from 1970 to 1980 the teenage birth rate fell by two fifths as contraception and sex education improved. Only one seventh of the decline was due to abortion (Francome 1983). In countries such as Russia and the Ukraine, contraceptive services have improved in recent years and abortion has become less common.

They Say Women should not be able to have an abortion or use modern methods of contraception even if there is a certainty that the resulting child would be severely handicapped. To quote the 'Declaration on Abortion' ratified by the Pope on 28 June 1974:

> A Christian (Catholic) outlook cannot be limited to the horizon of life in this world. He (sic) knows that during the present life another one is being prepared, one of such importance that it is in this light that such judgments must be made. From this viewpoint there is no absolute misfortune here below, not even the terrible sorrow of bringing up a handicapped child. This is the contradiction proclaimed by the Lord: 'happy those who mourn: They shall be comforted'.

Some people may wish to take the risk of producing a severely disadvantaged child and to bring it up in the best way possible. They should, of course, have the total support of the community and society should do whatever it can to provide help. However, there are many people who would have great difficulty in looking after such a child and these people should have the right to choose their method of fertility control.

Anti abortionists argue there should be no stem cell research to help the victims of Alzheimer's disease. On 26 November 2006 the Pope reiterated that he would never cease to warn of 'ethical problems of embryonic stem cell research'. US President George Bush took a similar view. However, in 2002 he was opposed by former President's wife Nancy Reagan. One observer called her 'one of the most revered icons of the Republican Party' and she was quoted as saying on the subject 'A lot of time is being wasted' (Francome 2004, p. 94).

Anti-abortionists often argue life begins at conception. In 1972 the Catholic Bishops of Massachusetts argued that there was no essential difference between an embryo and a starting quarterback in American football or a opera singer (Baird and Francome 1978). However, life does not begin at conception. Life begins pre-conception. Fertile people of both sexes contain the necessary means within them to procreate. However, if there is not live sperm and live eggs before conception then a pregnancy will not follow. Life is a continuous process not a singular event.

Unsafe Abortion is a Preventable Tragedy

There are many more deaths from unsafe abortion than there are from terrorism. However, the issues gets far less attention. This must lead us to conclude childbirth in general and abortion in particular are neglected problems of health care. The suffering is mainly in the developing countries. The moral and religious arguments around abortion have continued to obscure its importance as a serious public health problem. As a result successful policies and strategies to reduce the unnecessary numbers of deaths resulting from unsafe abortion have not been adopted.

Following the International Conference on Population and Development (ICPD) the abortion issue has received much more attention, a lack of reliable information and data on this problem has hampered a number of activities that would have helped to ameliorate the situation.

Illegal Abortion: The Colonial Legacy

When the rich countries such as France, Britain, Spain and the Netherlands colonized vast areas of the world they introduced new restrictive laws on the availability of contraception and abortion. These countries then legalized abortion on request at least in the early months of pregnancy. To do so the countries were sufficiently developed that they were able to disobey the dictates of the Catholic Church so that we have seen that even Italy the heart of the Catholic world now provides safe abortions to its women.

However, the colonists left the poorer countries with laws drafted largely in the nineteenth century. Furthermore, they left a situation where the former colonies were not able to assert their rights to safe medical care. We have seen the power of the Catholic Church in Latin America where it has been able to frustrate decriminalization and has forced women into a position where they have had to seek unsafe operations.

Jamaica is a good case in point. The UK had the Offences against the Person Act (1861). Four years later Jamaica followed suit and had its own Offences Against the Person Act. Almost 50 years ago the people of the UK were able to overthrow the restrictive provisions of the Act. However, Jamaican pro-choice forces have not had the strength to do likewise.

Aiding the Poorer Countries

We discussed governments' aid to the poor countries in the Introduction. On 30 May 2007 President Bush announced that the US was to double spending combating HIV/AIDS in Africa and three countries elsewhere to $30 billion over five years. However, the reports said 'a significant part of the funds will be channelled to religious groups advocating abstinence until marriage and refusing to distribute condoms.' The evidence of this book is that abstinence does not work as a policy so it is to be hoped that Republications will realize this if and when they regain power.

I reported the case of two prostitutes fighting over a used condom which they aimed to recycle, both of whom were hoping to protect their health. Such women deserve our help to safeguard themselves. The developed countries should ensure that everyone in the poor countries has access to condoms either for free or at very low prices.

Other modern methods of contraception also need to be supported and the rich Governments to help women use the kind of contraception most convenient for them. Stan Henshaw writes:

> Few developing countries offer a complete range of contraceptive methods. Countries need female sterilization AND male sterilization AND IUD AND norplant AND pills AND patch AND ring AND condoms AND periodic abstinence because different couples have different needs. And services are needed for unmarried women and teenagers as well as others. (Francome and Vekemans 2007)

Time to Change Laws

The abortion debate has focused largely on the moral issues of the value of the embryo or foetus in relation to the rights of women to control their bodies and the rights of couples to limit their childbearing. Our concern here, however, is with the public health consequences of various abortion policies, and the recommendations are for policies that best promote the health of women and children.

From a public health point of view, universal access to abortion services is clearly desirable. As explained, access to legal abortion has benefits for the health of both women and children. Thus, all restrictions that have the effect of reducing the supply of abortion providers or creating barriers for women seeking services are undesirable from the point of view of public health and welfare. There is little if any health justification for restricting abortion services that do not apply equally to other types of health care. Public health services in developing countries should cover abortion, since low-income women have the most need and face the greatest health risk from unwanted pregnancies. In almost all industrialized countries, government-sponsored health insurance covers abortion.

Canada provides evidence that no abortion-specific regulations are needed. The country has had no abortion law since 1988 with no ill effects on the health of women and with no excessive elevation of the abortion rate, which is lower than the rate in the US.

Legislation requiring special counselling for abortion, waiting periods, and parental involvement for minors serves no real purpose. If anything, women contemplating abortion need less special consideration than those planning to continue their pregnancies, since the risks and consequences of birth are greater than those of abortion. The medical community has perceived no need for regulations specific to women seeking prenatal care, and the same reasoning should apply to women seeking to terminate their pregnancies.

As in all fields of medicine, there are some physicians who provide sub-standard care and who exploit certain population groups, for example, by charging excessive fees to immigrants. There is no evidence, however, that licensing requirements specific to abortion improve the quality of care, while it is inevitable that such requirements increase costs and reduce the number of providers, thereby making it more difficult for women to gain access to abortion services. So the answer is to change restrictive laws and improve women's care.

Education

What is clear from our analysis of the world situation is that there is no major country which has successfully persuaded its population to practice abstinence on a wide scale and for the long periods necessary in times when marriages are being delayed. There are, however, a number of countries where contraceptive and health education has been such that the rates of unwanted pregnancy and abortion are greatly diminished. We have seen that in many countries there have been strong opponents of contraception. This is true for such disparate places as India where some recommend yoga instead, to the US where some teach abstinence. I would maintain that the way forward is provide good quality information to all young people and then if a proportion choose to be sexually abstinent then they have a choice.

Even in more prosperous countries there are gaps in services leading to those such as England and Wales having abortion rates twice as high as some of its continental neighbours. Hayley Blackburn of the UK's Family Planning Association writes:

> All young people should receive high quality personal social and health education from an early age. Although the UK Government has acknowledged the role of high quality sex and relationships education in supporting efforts to reduce rates of unintended pregnancies and sexually transmitted infections, it is still not a statutory part of the curriculum at all key stages and is sadly lacking in some areas of the country. Some basic elements of human reproduction are included in the national science curriculum and there is a requirement to teach young people about HIV and sexually transmitted diseases at secondary school. (Personal communication)

The guidance varies between each country within the UK, which results in extremely patchy provision. Young people consistently report that the sex and relationships education they receive at school is too little, too late and too biological. To provide young people with the knowledge, skills and confidence to make informed choices about their own sexual health, education must start from an early age and should achieve a balance between the acquisition of:

- *Attitudes* – appreciation of difference; tolerance; openness about sex.
- *Skills* – negotiation; communication; assertiveness; personal skills; managing emotions and relationships; problem-solving skills; decision-making skills.
- *Knowledge* – puberty; the mechanics of sex, including the biological aspects; fertility and reproduction; contraception and sexually transmitted diseases; information about sexual orientation and sexuality.

To ensure the quality of sexual, relationship and education provision, it is vital that the professionals responsible for its delivery are adequately trained. Some teachers do not feel comfortable teaching this material and training is required to support them to deliver it. A certification scheme for Personal, Social and Health Education, which has been introduced for teachers and school nurses, is to be welcomed.

Time for Catholics to Change Even More

Christianity began as a religion of love. 'Love one another even as I have loved you'. The Catholic Church used to reflect this and for over a thousand years priests were able to marry and have families. The Church was tolerant of sexual behaviour as a normal part of life. However, changes occurred and the church deviated a great deal from the early teachings of Christianity. It opposed priests and nuns having sexual relationships Married priests were banned from 1123. The Church criticized sex even within marriage and opposed people using contraception. The Catholic Church is doing some important work, for example, in helping to reduce poverty, but its positive actions are being undermined by the Church setting up standards of sexual behaviour which are unattainable for most people and leads to social problems. The priesthood in particular has had great problems. One difficulty is child abuse committed by priests denied normal family life. In Boston in 2003 $157 million was paid out to victims of sex abuse by priests. In Los Angeles in 2007 a sum of £325 ($660) million was paid to victims (*Scotsman* 2007). There is a debate as to whether this phenomenon is due to celibacy (Terry 2011) However. there has been agreement that sexual abstinence is a factor in the shortage of priests in the richer countries. The number of priests in the US declined from 59,000 in 1975 to 39,000 in 2013 despite the fact that the number of Catholics increased by 17 million over the period. Other countries such as Germany have imported priests from India (Priest Shortage 2013).

The Church has changed and we can identify four distinct areas around sexuality and the process is ongoing. First is the acceptance of married priests if they became Catholics. This first took place in 1980 and became important when a number of Anglicans converted over the issue of women priests.

Secondly is the changed attitude towards condoms. This was presented in a book by Pope Benedict in 2010 leading to a headline 'Pope breaks ice on Catholic view on condoms' (Henegan 2010). The Pope thought through the issue from the position of Thomas Aquinas and took the view that it was acceptable for male prostitutes to protect themselves or their male partners against HIV with condoms. He did not give a ringing endorsement but thought that condoms could be the lesser evil. Once this decision was taken it does not make sense to ban heterosexual wives from using condoms. As Tom Henegan commented:

> Many Catholic theologians came to the same conclusion years ago and some priests in Africa privately advise this if the alternative is infection, for example to a woman whose HIV-positive husband demands sex. (2010)

The dual purchase of condoms in both protecting against sexually transmitted diseases and pregnancy has been problematical for both the Church and the State. In Massachusetts in 1968 Bill Baird sat in prison for a month for giving a single woman contraceptive foam. He was not slow to point out that condoms were openly on sale in the State which was happy to collect its sales tax (personal communication). It was only legal to buy condoms for health protection until the U.S. Supreme Court overthrew the law in 1972 on the grounds of personal freedom (*Baird v Bellotti*). It paved the way for the abortion decision the following year.

Pope Francis

The successor to Pope Benedict has impressed a number of people by a more humanitarian approach. He has said that the church was too focused on preaching about abortion, gay people and contraception and needed to become more merciful. He also said 'If someone is gay and seeks the Lord with good will who am I to judge' (Kington 2014).

In November 2013 the Vatican sent out questionnaires to Catholic parishes. It resulted in a study of 12,000 Catholics worldwide being carried out in 12 countries. These countries between them hosted 6 out of ten of the global number of 1.2 billion Catholics. A BBC report commented 'Catholics around the world are more liberal than the Vatican' (BBC News 2014). The results found that on the issue of contraception the world's lay Catholics were more or less united against Church teaching. Over 90 per cent of the population were in favour of contraception in Argentina, Colombia, Brazil, Spain and France. The overall average was 78 per cent in favour. In the US it was 79 per cent and in the Philippines it was 68 per cent in support. Countries with the two low rates were both poorer – Congo 44 per cent and Uganda 43 per cent. Inglehart commented that the results showed:

> The less developed world is staying true to old world values, but it is gradually eroding ever there. (Pope Francis) doesn't want to lose the legitimacy of the more educated people.

On the issue of abortion the question asked 'Do you think abortions should be allowed in all cases, some cases such as when the life of the mother is in danger or should not be allowed at all' The results showed that nine per cent said abortion should be legal in all cases, 57 per cent said it should be legal in some cases and one third (33 per cent) said that it should not be allowed. There are problems with this type of question as I pointed out 30 years ago (Francome 1984, p. 215). However, it does seem to show that at least two thirds of Catholics oppose the total ban which is the official teaching.

In response to the results, Pope Francis has called for a rare 'extraordinary synod' in Autumn 2014 which will be on the topic 'The pastoral challenge of the family' (Inglehart 2014).

Pope Francis also seems to have shown a warm side to his personality in his comments about breastfeeding. Italian society has largely discouraged breastfeeding in public. However, in January 2014 the Pope broke with tradition and the news headline was 'Pope urges breastfeeding in Sistine chapel' It makes sense that nursing mothers do not have to take hungry children out of a service but rather can quietly nurse them (Sky News 2014).

Bring Abortion in from the Cold

We have seen that Catholic countries which discourage the use of modern methods of contraception tend to have high numbers of abortions. If abortion is illegal, it leads to unsafe operations. The proven way to reduce the number of abortions is to have good quality sex education, easy access to contraception and legal abortion at least in the early months of pregnancy. The Catholic Church can help facilitate this happening in two ways. First, it could change policy. The Church accepted abortion until 1869 and so it could revert to this position. In recent years it has espoused the doctrine that 'life begins at conception'. As mentioned above his doctrine is unsustainable as life begins before conception. Each fertile man and woman carries around with them the seeds of the future generation. With the average man carrying around 200 million live sperm only the smallest minority of these seeds will result in a live baby.

So if the Catholic Church is genuine about wishing to reduce the number of abortions it should support the policies of those countries with low abortion rates. These are the countries of Europe with good contraceptive facilities which give women the right to choose in the early months of pregnancy. However, even without changing policy it could follow the way of the Catholic Priest Father Robert Drinan in Massachusetts. He was also a US Member of Congress and Dean at the Boston Law College. He took the view that it was not good for the law to make decisions as to which foetuses should be born. Rather there should be a repeal of the law:

> One way to avoid the necessity of making these choices would be for the law to withdraw its protection from all fetuses during the first twenty-six weeks of their

> existence. Under this arrangement the law would not be required to approve or disapprove the choices of parents and physicians as to who may be born or not born. (Francome 1984, p. 113)

This position is more or less that of most Democratic presidential hopefuls in the US. They take the view that, while they personally may not agree with abortion, the law should not try to impose their morality. If the Catholic Church were to take this line it could keep to its position but help avoid the health problems that occur when abortion is criminalized.

As education develops the childbearing age is tending to rise and so the problem of age infertility is increasing. Some of these women can be helped by in-vitro fertilization; others whose partners are infertile may be helped by artificial insemination by donor. So far these aids to fertility have been opposed by the Church but a change of policy towards non-intervention or approval could help many women who hitherto have not received support.

So a change in policy by the Church could lead to great improvement in the health of society and aid family life.

Conclusion

The country by country analysis of this book has shown that abortion cannot be legislated out of existence. It is time for a more realistic approach to the whole area of sexuality and for action to stop the many silent deaths of women. All the countries of the world have a large part to play to improve health care for pregnant women. We have seen that maternal mortality rates are much too high especially in the poorer countries. It is time for women and mothers to enjoy good quality care.

Bibliography

Acosta, D. (2007) 'Many women prefer abortion to condoms', *Inter Press Service Agency.* <ipsnews.net/news.asp?idnews=33458> (Accessed 24 July 2007).

Action Now (2012) 'Yemen: End child marriage' *Equality Now*.

Advertisement (2013) available at: http:/bangaloregenesishospital.com/abortion-in-haiti.

AFP (2013) 'Aborton rights under attack, UN linked task force warns', afp@abortion.bling (Accessed 22 August 2013).

Akin, A., Kocoglu, G.O. and Akin, L. (2005) 'Study supports the introduction of early medical abortion in Turkey', *Reproductive Health Matters* 13(26).

Mturi, AJ. and Kembo, J. (2011) 'Falling fertility and increased use of contraception in Zimbabwe', *African J. of Reproductive Health* 5(2).

Al Sheeha M. (2010) 'Awareness and use of contraception amongst Saudi Women', *Int J Health Sci* (1):11–21.

Amagee, L.K. (1999) 'Recours a l'avortement provoque en milieu scolaire au Togo', Paper presented at International Seminar on 'Reproductive Health in Africa', Abidjan, Côte d'Ivoire.

Amnesty International (2013) 'Amnesty urges Chile rape victim's abortion rethink', BBC News.

Anderson, B. (2012) 'Anti-abortion activists protest in Panama City', 8 October, Channel 7 News.

Anderson, H. (1980) 'Abortion in Spain', *Peace News*, 25 January.

Anonymous (2013) 'Abortion in Mumbai', Under pseudonym Sarah. abortioninindia.com (Accessed 1 October).

Arabiya (2012) 'Saudi Clerics to mull whether Syrian women could abort a pregnancy from rape', 11 June, Al Arabiya. English@alarabiya.net (Accessed 10 December 2012).

Arilha, M. and Barbosa, R.M. (1993) 'Cytotec in Brazil', *Reproductive Health Matters* 1(21): 415–22.

Arthur, J. (1999) 'Legal abortion the sign of a civilised society', www.prochoiceactionnetwork.-Canada.org.civilised.htm (Accessed 17 July 2007).

Asami, E. (2013). 'Misunderstanding of law drives young women to self induced abortion in Ghana', 15 March, Ghana News Desk.

Asia News (2013) 'Nepal Medical Association against abortion', K. Parajuli (contact).

Austveg, B. and Sunby, J. (2005) Norway at ICPD+10. *Reproductive Health Matters* 13(25): 233.

Badgeley, R.F., Caron, N. and Powell, M.G. (1977) *Committee on the Operation of the Abortion Law.* Ministry of Supply and Services Canada, Ottawa.
Bailey, P.E. et al. (1988) 'A hospital study of illegal abortion in Bolivia', *Bulletin of the Pan American Health Organization* 22(1): 27–41.
Baranik, L. (2006) *Contraception and Abortion in the Czech Republic.* Expats CZ. www.expats.cz/prague/article/health-medical/contraception-abortion (Accessed 5 October 2013).
Barret, J. and Buckley, C. (2007) 'Constrained Contraceptive Choice: IUD prevalence in Uzbekistan', *International Family Planning Perspectives* 33(2): 507. www.guttmacher.org/pubs/journals/3305007.html.
BBC News (2012) 13 March, www.bbc.co.uk/news/world-latin-america-17360739.
BBC News (2014) www.bbc.co.uk/news/world/-europe=24821843.
BBC News (2012) 'Uruguay Legalises Abortion', 17 October.
Belton, S. et al. (2009) 'Maternal Mortality, Unplanned Pregnancy and Unsafe Abortion in Timor Leste', Alola Foundation. www.alolafoundation.org (Accessed 10 May 2013).
Berer, M. (2008) 'Why medical abortion is important to women', *Reproductive Health Matters* 13 (26) 6–10.
Biney, A.A.E (2011) 'Exploring contraceptive knowledge and use amongst women experiencing induced abortion in the greater Accra region of Ghana. *African J. of Reproductive Health* 15(1): 37–47.
Birkett, W.N. (1939) *Report of the Inter-Departmental Committee on Abortion.* London: HMSO.
Birth Rate Commission (1917) *The Declining Birth Rate 2nd edn.* London: Chapman and Hall.
Birthright (2011) 'Guatemala country program', swilliamsjd@wordpress.com/2011/04/18/birthright (Accessed 10 December 2013).
Blandine, T. (2012) 'Oral misoprostol as the first line care for incomplete abortion in Burkina Faso', *Int J of Gynaecology and Obstetrics* 119(2): 166–9.
Blandon, M.M. (2013) 'Abortion in El Salvador', by K. Zabudovsky and G. Palembo entitled 'Salvadoran Court Denies Abortion to Ailing Woman', *New York Times*, 29 May.
Bloom, M. (2008) 'Safe abortion hotline launched in anti-choice Ecuador', *Women on Waves*. 17 July.
Bonnefoy, P. (2009) 'Chile's Abortion Debate', *Global Press*, 3 February.
Boseley, S. (2011) 'Families increasingly aborting baby girls', *Guardian*, 24 May.
Brodie, J.S., Gavigan, A.M. and Jenson, J. (1992) *The Politics of Abortion.* Toronto: Oxford University Press.
Brodzinsky, S. (2006) 'Church condemns abortion carried out on raped girl eleven', *The Guardian* 31 August.
Brook, J. (2002) 'N. Koreans talk of baby killings' www.ibtimes.co.uk/north-korea-human-rights-united-nations-516329.
Brookman-Amissah, E. (2013) 'Abortion law in sub-Saharan Africa: no turning back', www.ncbi.nlm.gov/pubmed/15938178 (Accessed 9 October 2013).

Bumwe, R. (2012) 'Religion, Confusion on Rwanda's New Abortion Drive Debate', *Global Press Institute*, 6 November.

Burcombe, A. (2005) 'Colombian Abortion Law Campaign', 13 October. *The Independent.*

Bury, L. and Ngo, T.D. (2009) *The condom broke! Why do women in the UK have unintended pregnancies?* London: MSI.

Cabatu, E. and Bonk, K. (2005) 'Media summary', *Agence France Presse*, 6 March.

Caeser, M. (2006) 'Court ends Colombia abortion ban', *The Lancet* 367(9523): 16–45.

Canadian Institute for Health Information (2014) http://www.cihi.ca/cihi-ext-portal/pdf/internet/ta 11 alldatatables2013o221 (Accessed 21 June 2014).

Can/LW News (2007) 'Uruguay's new top judge backs abortion', CAN/LW News. 1 February.

Caribbean Catholic (2012) 'Looking at the world', 29 May.

Cartoof, V.G. and Klerman, L.V. (1986) 'Parental consent for abortion: impact of the Massachusetts law', *Am J of Public Health* 76(4): 397–400.

Cathcart, A. (2012) 'Prostitution, abortion and flower girls: women in Hyesan', www.sinonk.com/2012/08/02/prostitution-abortion-Hyesan-north-korea (Accessed 9 October 2013).

Catholic News Agency (2009) 'President of Honduras gives green light to morning after pill', Press Release, 20 May, Tegucigalpa www.Catholicnewsagency (Accessed 11 December 2013).

Catholic Poll (2014) www.washingtonpost.com/wp-srv/spwcial/worldcatholic/poll.

Catlinotti, E. (2007) 'Portugal', *Worker's World*, 13 February.

Centre for Reproductive Rights (2005) *The World's Abortion Laws*. http://www.crlp.org/pub_fac_abortion_laws.html. (Accessed 11 November 2013).

Centre for Reproductive Rights (2007) *The World's Abortion Laws.* Briefing paper, July.

Centre for Reproductive Rights (2011) 'Nepal Supreme Court: Abortion is a Right'.

Centre for Reproductive Rights (2012) 'Rwanda: Government takes Critical Step in Recognizing Women's Rights', 15 August. www.reproductiverights.org./en/feature/need-to-reform-in-rwanda. (Accessed 3 March 2013).

Centre for Reproductive Rights (2012a) *Honduras Supreme Court Upholds Absolute Ban on Emergency Contraception.*

Chakwe, M. (2013) 'Birth Control Use in Zambia Relatively Low', 22 April.

Charles, J. (2013) 'Abortion in Haiti: Dangerous and Illegal', 5 December. Television transcript, http//kacu.org/post/abortion-haiti-dangerous-and-illegal.

Chelela, C. (1998) 'Algerian abortion controversy highlights rape of war victims', *Lancet* 351: 1413.

Childbirth by Choice Trust (1998) *No Choice: Canadian Women Tell their Stories of Illegal Abortion.* Toronto: Childbirth by Choice.

Chinoy, M. (2007) 'Vietnam's High Abortion Rate', *Medical News Today*, 18 February.

Choike (2002) *Women and Health in Uruguay*, www.choike.org (Accessed 10 December 2006.

CNA (2013) www.catholicnewsagency.com/news/un-harshly-criticised-for-pushing-abortion-in-peru/. (Accessed 2 April 2013).

Cohen, N. (2012) 'Bolivia's Clandestine Abortion Industry', *Bolivian Express*, 14 August.

Conde, C.H. (2005) 'Philippines Abortion Crisis', *International Herald Tribune* 16 May.

COPUA (2013) http://www.nyasatimes.com/2013/10/18/malawi-abortion-law-needs-reform-copua (Accessed 18 October 2013)

CRR (2011) Reproductive rights.org/en/press-room/un-rules-that-peru-must-relax-restriction-on-abortion. 11 July.

Cunningham, E. (2013) 'Where is the worst place for abortions?', *Global Post* January.

De Silva, W.I. (2003) *Reproductive Health in Sri Lanka*, US Aid. www.ncbi.nlm.nih.gov/pmc/articles/pmc2386785. (Accessed 8 October 2013).

De Bruin, J. (1979) *Geschiedennis van abortus in Nederland.* Amsterdam: Van Gennep.

DeJong, J., Jawad, J., Mortagy, I. and Shepard, B. (2005) 'The sexual and reproductive behaviour of young people in the Arab countries and Iran', *Reproductive Health Matters* 13(25):49–50.

Del Carmen, Elu M. (1993) 'Abortion Yes, Abortion No in Mexico', *Reproductive Health Matters* (1): 58–66.

DeMarchi, L. (no date) 'Bringing contraception to Italy: A story of moral heroism', Published by *Church and State.*

De Sam Lazero, F. (2004) *Religion and Ethics*, newsletter www.pbs.org/newshour/bb/africa/janjune04zambia.01-08html (Accessed 9 January 2007).

De Sam Lazero, F. (2011) 'Brazil's shifting views of Church, abortion and lifestyle', 30 August, PBS Newshour, http//wwwpbs.org/newshour/rundown/2011/08/Brazil-abortion.html.

Deschner, A. and Cohen, S.A. (2003) 'Contraceptive use is key to reducing abortion'. New York: Guttmacher Institute.

Diagne, B. (2012) 'Abortion an illegal and secret practice in Senegal', Radio Netherlands Worldwide. http://www.allafrica.com/dtores/201202011137.html.

Dosybieva, O. (2005) 'Kazakstan:illegal abortion concerns count', http://www.jwpr.net/index.pl?archive/rca2 366 2 eng.txt (Accessed 26 June 2013).

Downie, A. (2010) 'Abortions in Brazil, though illegal, are common', http//content.time.com/time/world/article/0.8599.1993205.html.

Drummond, K. (2010) 'Afghan Mullahs Promote birth control to save lives', AOL News, 2 March.

Duffy, G. (2007) 'Brazil to subsidise contraception', http//news.bbc.co.uk/i/hi/world/Americas/6699719.stm, 27 May.

Easton, A. (2007) 'Polish woman wins abortion case', BBC News, Warsaw. http://news.bbc.co.uk (Accessed 4 April 2007).

Editorial (2011) 'Legal abortion in Thailand unlikely', *Thailand Times* 29 May.

Education for Choice (2013) personal communication.

Egan, J.E., Benn, P.A., Zelop, C.M. et al. [DATE] 'Down syndrome births in the United States 1989–2001', *Am J of Obstetrics and Gynaecology* 191(3):1044–8.

El Damanhoury, H. (2013) 'Abortion is illegal and common in Egypt', www.medicalabortionconsortium.org/uploads/file/Egypt.pdf (Accessed 2 October 2013).

Ellis, H.H. (1928) *Psychology of Sex*. London: Heinemann.

Erfani, A. (2011) 'Induced abortion in Tehran, Iran: estimates of rates and correlates', *International Perspectives on Sexual and Reproductive Health* 37(3).

Ertelt, S. (2012) 'Costa Rico ban on IVF defended in court', LifeNews.com 5 August.

Estrada, D. (2006) 'Chile: Therapeutic abortion a distant but not impossible prospect', psnews.net.net/news.asp?idnews=34850 (Accessed 17 July 2007).

EWTN News (2007) 'Abortion ban a crime', 3 August.

EWTN News (2011) 'Report finds abortion is 'getting out of hand' in Cuba' (Accessed 13 March 2015).

Faundes, A., Duarte, G.A., Neto, J.A. and de Souza, M.H. (2004) 'The closer you are the better you understand: the reaction of Brazilian obstetrican-gynaecologists to unwanted pregnancy. *Reproductive Health Matters* 12(24):47–56.

Fargues, P. (2005) 'Women in Arab countries: challenging the patriarchal system', *Reproductive Health Matters* 13(25): 43–8.

Fernandez, P. (2013) 'Uruguayan Abortion Law will not go to referendum', www.ewtnnews.org/catholic-news/us.phpd= (Accessed 2 October 2013).

Fetters, S.T. (2012) 'Abortion care needs in Darfur and Chad', *Forced Migration Review*, 3 May. Connection.ebscohost.com/…/22181031 (Accessed 22 May 2013).

Finney, P.A. (1935) *Moral Problems in Hospital Practice 5th edn.* New York: B. Herder Book Company. New York.

Fonseca, H. and Pujol, P. (2004) 'A Drama Unfolds', *New Internationalist*. November.

Francome, C. and Vekemans, M. (2007) *Abortion: A Worldwide Perspective*. London: Middlesex University Press.

Francome, C. (1976) 'How many illegal abortions', *British J. of Criminology* October.

Francome, C. (1984) *Abortion Freedom*. Hemel Hempstead: Unwin Hyman.

Francome, C. (1986) *Abortion Practice*. Hemel Hempstead: Unwin Hyman.

Francome, C. (2000) *Karl Marx: Hero or Zero*. London: Carla Publications.

Francome, C. (2004) *Abortion in the USA and the UK*. Aldershot: Ashgate Publishing Ltd.

Friedman-Rudovsky, J. (2007) 'Abortion under Siege in Latin America', *La Paz* 9 August. www.content time.com/time/world/article/0.8599.1651307.00.html (Accessed 5 October 2013).

Fuchs, D. (2005) 'Spanish abortion rate soars', *Guardian* 28 December.

Gabbat, A. (2012) 'Jamaican Doctor arrested for performing an abortion on a twelve year old', *Guardian* 13 July.

Gallo, M.F., Gebresclassie, H., Victorino, M.T.A. et al., (2004) 'Assessment of abortion facilities in public health facilities in Mozambique: women's and providers Perspectives' *Reproductive Health Matters* 12(24): 218–26.

Ganatra, B., Bygdeman, M., Thuy, et al. (2004) 'From research to reality: the challenges of introducing medical abortion into service in Vietnam' *Reproductive Health Matters* 12(24): 105–13.

Genethique (2005) www.genethique.org (Accessed 14 July 2007).

Girard, F. (2012) realitycheck.org/article/2012/12/19/double-jeopardy-rape-victims-in-peru/, 19 December.

Giovanni, J. (2012) 'After the Arab spring Yemen's women are left behind', http://www.newsweek.com/after-arab-spring-yemens-women-are-left-behind-63457 (Accessed 17 March).

The Gleaner (2012), 'Abortion for sale – black market thrives on baby killing pills'. http://jamaicanewsonline.com/jamaicagleaner/abortion-for-sale-black-market-thrives-on-baby-killing-pills/ (Accessed 6 May).

Govan, F. (2009) 'Spain prepares to fully legalize abortion', *Daily Telegraph* 20 February.

Grimes, D.A., Benson, J., Singh, S. et al. (2006) 'Unsafe Abortion the Preventable Pandemic', www. medicalnewstoday.com/articles/55593php (Accessed 22 May 2013).

Gutierrez, E. (2010) 'Abortion in Latin America-still illegal, still killing people', *Upside Down World.*

Guttmacher Institute (2006) *State Policies in Brief: State Funding of Abortion under Medicaid.* New York: Guttmacher Institute.

Guttmacher Institute (2008) *Abortion in Indonesia.* New York: Guttmacher Institute.

Guttmacher Institute (2010) *Facts on Unintended Pregnancy and Abortion in Ethiopia*. New York: Guttmacher Institute.

Guttmacher Institute (2012) *Facts on Abortion in Latin America and the Caribbean.* New York: Guttmacher Institute.

Guttmacher Institute (2012a) *Facts on Abortion in Africa.* New York: Guttmacher Institute.

Guttmacher Institute (2013) *Facts on Induced Abortion Worldwide.* http://www.Guttmacher.org/pubs/fb_IAW.html. (Accessed 28 August).

Guttmacher Institute (2014) *State Policies in Brief: Parental Involvement in Minors' Abortions*. New York: Guttmacher Institute.

Guttmacher Institute (2014a) *State Policies in Brief: Counseling and Waiting Periods for Abortion.* New York: Guttmacher Institute.

Gumbel, A. (2006) 'Colombia ruling breaks seal on abortion', *Independent* 13 May.

Guttmacher, S., Kapadia, F. et al. (1998) 'Abortion law reform in South Africa: a case study of the 1996 Choice of Termination of Pregnancy Act', *International Family Planning Perspectives* 24(4).

Gyimah, S.O. (2011) 'Ghanaian Family Planning Policy', *Think Africa Press*, 20 October.

Gynuity (2012) gynuity.org/locations/country/Guatemala (Accessed 17 March).

Hajnal, J. (1965) 'A Comparison of Family Patterns in Eastern and Western Europe'. in Glass, D.V. and Eversley, D.E.C. (eds), *Population in History*. London: Methuen.

Halkias, A. (2005) *Greek American Review*. March, pp. 24–8.

Hall, K.G. (2003) 'Abortion in Brazil: a debate divided along moral and class lines', *Knight Ridden Newspapers*, 28 July.

Harvey, S. (2014) 'Abortion rate lowest for twenty years', http://www.staff.co.nz/national/health/9577045/ab-rate.

Hayes, J. (2011) 'Birth control in Japan', Internet facts and details.com/japan.php?itemid=599.

Heneghan, T. (2010) http://blogs.reuters.com/faithword/2010/11/21analysis.

Hennesy, M. and Smyth, J. (2007) 'European ruling in Polish abortion case can affect the law here', *Irish Times*, 21 March.

Henshaw, S.K. and Kost (1992) 'Parental involvement in minor's abortion decisions', *Family Planning Perspectives* 24(5): 196–207.

Henshaw, S.K., Singh, S. and Hass, T. (1999) 'The incidence of abortion worldwide', *Family Planning Perspectives* 25 (Supplement) January.

Henshaw, S. (1995) 'The impact of requirement for parental consent on minors abortions in Mississippi', *Family Planning Perspectives* 27(3): 120–2.

Hessini, L. (2007) 'Abortion and Islam: policies and practice in the Middle East and North America', *Reproductive Health Matters* 15(29): 75–84.

Hitt, J. (2006) 'Pro-life nation', *New York Times* 9 April.

Hirve, S.S. (2004) 'Abortion law policy and services in India: a critical review', *Reproductive Health Matters* 12(24): 114–21.

Holland, K. (2012) 'Savita Halappanavar's death may stir Ireland to change over abortion', *The Observer*, 17 November.

Human Rights Watch (2005) 'Help for the victims', hrw.org/reports/2005/drc0305/8. (Accessed 17 March 2015).

Human Rights Watch (2007a) 'Women's Rights', chile.hrw.org (Accessed 17 June).

Human Rights Watch (2007b) 'Women's Rights: Columbia' Colombia.hrw.org/English/docs/2995/6/22/colomb (Accessed 17 July).

Human Rights Watch (2007d) 'Mexico: Rape victims denied legal abortion rights', hrw.org/English docs 2006/2/23/mexico (Accessed 17 July).

Hussein, R. (2012) *Abortion and unintended pregnancy in Kenya*. Guttmacher Institute Factsheet. May, New York.

Illingworth, B. (2006) 'Mexico's abortion law', Planned Parenthood of the USA New York. www.pp.org//politics-policy-issues/international-issues/mexico-abortion-13045.ntm (Accessed 24 July 2007).
Index Mundi (2013) 'Contraceptive prevalence in Iraq', www.indexmundi.com/facts/Iraq/contraceptive-prevalence (Accessed 2 October 2013).
Index Mundi (2014) indexmundi.com/facts/Guyana/unmet-need-for-contraception
International Campaign (2013a) 'Unsafe abortions continue in Kenya despite reforms', 30 August. Information by email.
International Campaign (2013b) personal information.
International Campaign (2014) http//:www.change.org/en-GB/petitions/the–un-secretary-general-make-women-matter.
International Women's Health Coalition (2007) 'Abortion in Peru', www.Nytimes/gst/fullpage.html?res9DOOE1DF (Accessed 17 July).
Inter Press Service (2004) 'Health: Nigerian Abortion law takes a toll', www.ipsnews.net/2004/08 (Accessed 10 April).
Ioonnide-Kapolou, E. (2004) 'Use of contraception and abortion in Greece: a review', *Reproductive Health Matters* 12(24): 174–83.
IPPF (2013) *Abortion Sri Lanka.* International Planned Parenthood Federation London.
IPPF (2014) www.org/our-work/where-we-work/western-hemisephere.
IRIN Asia (2013) 'Timor Leste: abortion laws in the spotlight', www.irinnews.org (Accessed 15 February).
IRIN (2009) 'Health' Irin online 15 March. www.irinnews.org (Accessed 10 November 2012).
IRIN (2010) Burma www.irinnews.org//report88383/myanmar-abortion-a-leading-cause-of-maternal-death (Accessed 2 February 2014).
IRIN (2010a) Myanmar, www.irinnews.org (Accessed 20 February 2012).
IRIN (2011) 'Nigeria: changing attitudes to contraception' www.irinnews.org (Accessed 27 July 2913).
IRIN (2012) 'Boosting contraceptive use to cut unsafe abortions', www.irinnews.org (Accessed 21 April 2013).
IRIN (2012a) 'South Sudan: contraceptives give women the right to choose'. www.irinnews.org (Accessed 20 March 2013).
IRIN (2012B) 'Menstrual medication with medication', *Medical abortion matters.* www.irinnews.org (Accessed January 2013).
IRIN (2013) 'Concern over unsafe abortion in Papua New Guinea', www.irinnws.org (Accessed 20 July 2013).
Genethique (2005) www.genethique.org (Accessed 14 July 2007).
Jacobson, J. (2012) 'Honduras Supreme Court upholds most sweeping ban on emergency contraception', *RH Reality Check*, 14 February.
Jaffer, N. (2012) 'Unprotected sex in South Sudan', *The Guardian*, 30 May.
Jagwe-Wadda, G., Moore, A.M. and Wong, V. (2006) *Abortion Morbidity in Uganda*. New York: Guttmacher Institute.
Jahani, F. (2004) 'Abortion in Iranian Law', *Iranian Daily*, 15 January.

Jiyeon, A. (2008) 'Illegal abortion South Korea's open secret', *Reuters*, 4 April.

Johnson, B.R., Horga, M. and Fajans, P. (2004) 'A strategic assessment of abortion and contraception in Romania', *Reproductive Health Matters* 12(24): 184–94.

Johnston, W.R. (2013) *Historical Abortion Statistics: Israel*, www.johnstonarchive.net (Accessed 27 February 2014).

Johnston, W.R. (2013b*) Historical Abortion Statistics: Japan*, www.Johnstonarchive.net (Accessed 10 August 2014).

Johnston, W.R. (2013c) *International Encyclopaedia of Sexuality. Italy*, www.johnstonarchive.net (Accessed 19 July).

Johnston, W.R. (2013d) *Historical Abortion Statistics: Norway*, www.Johnstonarchive.net (Accessed 1 October).

Johnston, W.R. (2013e) *Historical Abortion Statistics: Ukraine*, www.johnstonarchive.net (Accessed 10 July).

Johnston, W.R. (2013f) *Historical Abortion Statistics: Kazakhstan*, www.johnstonarchive.net (Accessed 26 August).

Johnston, W.R. (2013g) *Historical Abortion Figures: Vietnam*, www.johnstonarchive.net (Accessed 17 July).

Johnston W.R. (2013h) *Historical Abortion Statistics: Sweden* www.johnstonarchive.net (Accessed 26 June 2014).

Johnston, W.R. (2013j) *Historical Abortion Statistics: New Zealand.* www.johnstonarchive.net (Accessed 10 June 2013).

Johnston W.R. (2013k) *Historical Abortion Statistic: Russia.* www.johnstonarchive.net (Accessed 8 January 2013).

Johnston W.R. (2013L) *Historical Abortion Statistics: Romania* www.johnstonarchive.net (Accessed 14 January 2013).

Johnston W.R. (2013m) *Historical Abortion Statistics: Spain.* www.johnstonarchive.net (Accessed 25 January 2013).

Johnston W.R. (2013n) *Historical Abortion Statistics: Uzbekistan* www.johnstonarchive.net (Accessed 3 March 2013).

Jones R.K., Darrach, J.E. and Henshaw, S. (2002) 'Patterns in the socioeconomic characteristics of women obtaining abortions in 2000–2001', *Perspectives on Sexual and Reproductive Health* 34(5): 226–35.

Joyce, T., Kaestner, R. and Coleman, S. (2006) 'Change in abortion and births and the Texas parental notification law', *New England J of Medicine* 354(10): 1031–8.

Juaraz, F. et al. (2005) 'The incidence of induced abortion in the Philippines', *International Journal of Family Planning Perspectives* 31(3) September.

Juaraz, F. et al. (2008) 'Estimates of illegal abortions in Mexico', *International Journal of Family Planning Perspectives* 34(4) December.

Kanyalika (2013) 'Malawi has 77,000 abortions', Malawi Voice, www.malawivoice.com/2013/3/27 (Accessed 10 September 2013).

Karafin, A. (2008) 'Tragic epidemic: Unsafe Abortion in Senegal', *Ms Magazine* 27 May, www.rhrealitycheck.org/article/2008/05/27/tragic-epidemic-unsafe-abortion-senegal.

Katzive, L. (2007) 'Law Changes 1996–2007', Centre for Reproductive Rights. New York.

Kestler, E. (2012) 'Obs/gynae new dosage for misoprostol from WHO', *International J of Gyn and Obs* 116(2) February.

Kington, T. (2014) www.news.nationalpost.com/2014/02/09/popes-global-survey-reveals-more-catholics-support-abortion-divorce-than-previously-thought.

Ketting, E. and Schnabel, P. (1980) 'Induced abortion in the Netherlands: a decade of experience', *Studies in Family Planning* 11(12): 385–94.

Kissoon, C. (2012) 'Pregnant little girl a case for abortion?', *Trinidad Express* 20 July.

Kitamura, K. (2005) 'Abortion' *Japan's Mental Health* 6 November.

Kristof, N. (2010) 'Poverty and the Pill', *New York Times* (OP ED) 19 May.

Kommers, D.P. (1977) 'Abortion and the Constitution: United States and West Germany', *Am J of Comparative Law* 25(2): 225–85.

Kotch, C.S. (2012) 'A ground breaking abortion study from Chile', Mercatornet. www.Mercatornet /…/abortion.gbasfe (Accessed 28 December 2012).

Lafaurie, M.M., Grossman, D., Troncoso, E., Billings, D.L. and Chavez, S. (2005) 'Women's perspectives on medical abortion in Mexico, Colombia, Ecuador and Peru: a qualitive study', *Reproductive Health Matters* 13(26): 75–83.

Larijani, B. and Zahedi, F. (2006) 'Changing parameters for abortion in Iran', *J of Medical Ethics*, www.Globalbioethics.blogspot.com/2007-03-01archive.html (Accessed 17 July 2007.)

Lautmann, R. and Starke, K. (2005) *International Encyclopaedia of Sexuality: Germany.* Published by Kinsey Institute.

Life Site News (2006) 'Muslims approve cloning in Malaysia' www.lifesite. net/idn/2003/jan (Accessed 4 April 2007).

Life Site News (2009) 'Honduras passes a law prohibiting abortifacient "emergency contraception"'. Press release, 7 April.

Linner, B, (1968) *Sex and Society in Sweden.* London: Jonathan Cape.

McLaran, A. and McLaran, M.T. (1997) *The Bedroom and the State: The Changing Practices and Politics of Contraception and Abortion in Canada, 1880–1997 2nd edn.* Oxford: Oxford University Press.

MacNevin, S. (2012) 'The Iraq Women's Rights Coalition', Internet. www.equalityinIraq.com (Accessed 27 September 2013).

McDonald, H. (2012) 'Ireland should change abortion law after woman's death', *The Guardian,* 14 November.

McGeown, K. (2011) 'Fierce Debate over Philippine Contraception Bill.' www.bbc.co.uk/news/world-asia-15822637 (Accessed 28 September 2013).

Majaj, Y. (ed.) (2005) *Ten Years after Beijing* New York: Arab NGOs UN Development Fund.

Makamure, L. (2012) 'Angola Abortion Bill Causes Uproar', South African Gender Protocol Alliance. www.genderlinks.org.za/article (Accessed 7 April 2013).

Make Every Woman Count (2011) *Africa: Maputo Protocol* (Updated March 2013). www.makeeverywomancount.org /…/id=892africa-maputo (Accessed 2 October 2013).

Martens, J. (2004) 'Congo rape victims seek solace', BBC News 24 January.

Meaney, J. (2003) 'A pro-life missionary trip', *Human Life International*, pp. 101–3.

Medina, A. (2012) Pro-life advocates warn of legalised abortion', EWTN News. www.ewtnnews.com/catholic-news/new.php.id=5663 (Accessed 5 October 2013).

Methodist Church (2003) 'Untitled discussion on the position of the Church in Uruguay' (Released 3 February).

Ministère de la Sante (2003) *Division de la Sante Familiale*. University of Lomé.

Montesinos, L. and Preciado, J. (2007) 'Abortion: Puerto Rico', *International Journal of Sexuality*, available at www.sexquest.com//esa/iesi-3contents.html (Accessed 17 July 2007).

Moore, C. (2013) 'Speech to the Senate', 26 February 2013 posted by *Sexual Health and the FPA*, Australia.

Moore, T. (2003) 'On board Poland's abortion ship', bbcwladyslawowo. www. newsbbc.co.uk /2/hi/europe/3051436.stm (Accessed 4 October 2013).

Moraes, T. (2011) 'Brazil's unsafe abortions impede development goal', http/ womanse.news.org/story/abortion/110915/Brazil's-unsafe-abortions-impede-development-goal (Accessed 18 January 2014).

MSI (2007a) *Sri Lanka* London: MSI.

MSI (2007b) *Uganda: Providing a lifeguard against HIV*. London: MSI.

MSI (2013) 'Nepal: New figures show safe abortion services', Contact, Tony Kerridge.

MSI (2013a) 'Where in the World: Madagascar' (Accessed 19 April 2013).www. mariesstopes.org/where-in-the=world/madagascar.

MSI (2013b) 'Where in the World: Yemen'. London: MSI.

Mundoandino: http://mundoandino.com/Argentina/Abortion-in-Argentina (Accessed 17 January 2014).

Mushabati, N. (2012) *Abortion in Zambia*, published by OSISA, www.osisa.org/ sites/default/files/19-24pdf (Accessed 25 April 2013).

Mturi, A.J. and Hinde, A. (2001) *Fertility levels and differentials in Tanzania* www. un.org/esa/population publications/prospects decline info3.pdf. (Accessed 30 April 2013).

Myers, S.L (2003) 'After decades Russia narrows grounds for abortion', *New York Times*, 24 August.

National Center for Health Statistics (2013) Data Brief Number 136.

Nelsen, A. (2013) 'Taking calls on abortion and risks in Chile', *New York Times*, 3 January.

Ngambi, R.N. (2005) 'A need to review the abortion laws in Belgium', www.enzinearticles.com/?a-need-to-review-abortion-articles-in-Belgium&id=39129 (Accessed 4 October 2013).

Nunes, F.E. and Delph, Y.M. (1995) 'Making Abortion Law Reform Happen in Guyana: A Success Story', *Reproductive Health Matters* 3(6): 12–23.

Nunes, F.E. (2012) 'Legal but inaccessible in Guyana', *Social and Economic Studies* 61(3): 59–94.

Nyasa Times (2012) 'Malawi promises to raise contraceptive prevalence rate to 60 per cent', *Nyasa Times* 12 July.

Nyasa Times (2013) 'Has Parliament legalised abortion? Malawi bishops condemn abortion in a pastoral letter', *Nyasa Times*, www.nyasatimes/com/2013/03/02/ (Accessed 10 September 2013).

O'Hanlon, E. (2013) 'Dynamics of abortion', 19 May, Information from International Campaign. (by email).

Okeowo, A. (2011) 'Africa's abortion wars', *International Herald Tribune*, 15 December.

Oliver Miller, S. (2004) http://www.kinseyinstitute.org/ccies/pg.php.

Olori, T. (2007) 'Abortion law takes a toll', *International Press News Agency* 15 February.

Olson (2013) www.koreabang.com/2013/stories/controversial-book-on-abortion-in-south-korea-triggers-debate.

Osofsky, H.J. and Osofsky, J.D. (1973) *The Abortion Experience.* New York: Harper and Row.

Ottoway, M. (2004) *Women's Rights and Democracy in the Arab World.* Washington, DC.

Ouattara, A. (2006) http://www.ipsnews.net/2006/08/health-cote-divoire-abortion-illegal-sought-after-sometimes-fatal/ (Accessed 17 March).

Oubliette, D. (2010) 'Is it safe to get an abortion in Egypt?', answers.yahoo.com/question/omdex?qid=20100503132751AAFIHEO, 3 May.

Oumar, C.Z. (2012) 'Côte d'Ivoire: contraception' *contraceptif voie*, 2 March.

Page, J. (2007) 'Hospital mass grave found as India cracks down on female infanticide', *The Times* 19 February, Sect 1: Sect 27(1).

Palmdoc (2006) 'Should abortion be legalised in Malaysia', *Malaysian Medical Resources* http/www.medicine.com.my/wp/wp-mobile.php?p=13288more=1 (Accessed 17 July 2007).

Parry, R.L. (2013) 'Spain hesitates on contentious abortion reform', AFP 9 June www.uk.news.yahoo.com/Spain-hesitates-controversial-abortion-reform (Accessed 4 June 2013).

Pangkahila, W. and Pangkahila, J.A. (2006) *Indonesia. www.2.* husberlin. de.sexuology /IES/Indonesia part 1.html (Accessed 17 June 2007).

Pathfinder (2012a) 'Introducing integrated mobile team to Burundi', www. pathfinder.org/publications-tools/introducing (Accessed 11 August 2013).

Paulson, K.D. (2007) Seventh-Day Adventists: Abortion (leaflet produced 17 April).

Paxman, J.M. (1980) *Law and Planned Parenthood.* London: IPPF.

Pelrine, V.W. (1972) *Abortion in Canada.* Toronto: New Press Toronto.

Perazza, T. (2008) 'Brazil and Vatican spar over abortion rights', http//womanse.news.org/story/reproductive-health/080201/brazil-and-vatican-spar-over-reproductive-rights.

Perlez, J. (2007) 'Warsaw bans a clinic's in-vitro fertilization treatments', *New York Times* 3 April.

Perner, R.A. (2007) *Austria: Reputik Osterreich International Encyclopedia of Sexuality*. www2.hu-berlin.de sexology/IES/Austria (Accessed 17 July 2007).

Pflanz, M. (2012) *Somalia approves Constitution*, 1 August. www.telegraph.co.uk (Accessed 3 October 2013).

Pheterson, G. and Azize, Y. (2005) 'Abortion practice in the NE Caribbean: just write down stomach pain', *Reproductive Health Matters* 13(26): 44–53.

Plank, E. (2013) 'France makes contraception and abortion free', *Politics* www.policymic.com (Accessed 6 October 2013).

Planned Parenthood (2012) 'Ecuador Country program', www.plannedparenthood.org/about-us/internationalprogram (Accessed 9 June 2013).

UN Population Division (2007a) *Abortion Policy: Yemen.* New York: Department of Economic and Social Affairs.

UN Population Division (2007b) *Abortion Policy: Zambia.* New York: Department of Economic and Social Affairs.

UN Population Division (2007c) *Abortion Policy: Uzbekistan.* New York: Department of Economic and Social Affairs.

Population Information Programme (2007) Centre for Communication Programmes 25(1). Johns Hopkins University.

Population Matters (2012) 'Tanzania: What about contraception', *Huffington Post* 7 October.

Population Policy (2011) *Venezuela.* www.un.org (Accessed 28 April 2013).

Population Policy (2013) *Kazakstan.* www.un.org (Accessed 17 June 2013).

Population Policy (2013a).

Potts, M., Diggory, P. and Peel, J. (1977) *Abortion.* Cambridge: Cambridge University Press.

Potts, M. et al. (2011) 'Niger: too little, too late' *International Perspectives on Sexual and Reproductive Health* 37(2) June.

PRI (2006) 'The epidemiology of abortion in pro-life Panama', www.un.org/esa/population/publications/abortion/doc/panama.doc.

Priest Shortage (2013) www.patheus.com/blogs/.../cbs-discover]the-catholic-priest-shortage.

Rapoza K (2013) 'Police raid Rio De Janeiro abortion Clinic', 6 January, ICSA.

Rasch, V. and Lyaruu, M.A. (2005) 'Unsafe abortion in Tanzania: the need for involving men in post abortion counselling', *Family Planning Perspectives* 36(4): 201–10.

RCOG (2008) 'Reasons to do away with two doctors signatures', May (updated 2010).

Religion and Ethics (2004) Newsletter, Zambia, 9 January.

Reynolds, M. (2005) 'Abortion rate drops to the lowest ever', *The Oreque Post* 27 July.

Rogers, J.L., Boruch, R.F., Stoms, G.B. et al. (1991) 'Impact of the Minnesota parental notification law on abortion and birth', *Am. J of Public Health* 81(3): 294–8.

Rossier, C., Guielle, G., Ouedraogo, A. and Thieba, B. (2004) 'Estimating clandestine abortion with the confidence method: Results from Ouagadougou, Burkina Faso'. Paper presented at the Population Association of America. April.

Ross, J. (2005) 'Illegal abortion rampant in Latin America', Women's News. www.womensnews.org.article.cfm/dyn/aid2086/context/archive (Accessed 15 September 2013).

Ross, J. (2006) 'Chile teens sex health', Women's News www.womensnews.org/article.cfm/dyn/aid/2895/context/archive (Accessed 17 July 2007).

Ross, W. (2010) 'DR Congo gang rape crisis is spreading, new study says', BBC News, 15 April.

Round up (2005) 'Health and health services suffering in Iraq', *Reproductive Health Matters* 13: 190.

Sai, F.T. (2011) 'Family Planning leaders should do more', *The Zimbabwean*, 17 November.

Schuster, S. (2005) 'Abortion in the moral world of the grass fields of Cameroon', *Reproductive Health Matters* 13(26): 130–8.

Scommegna, P. (2012) http://www.prb.org/publications/articles/2012/Morrocco-maternal-deaths-aspx.

Scotsman (2007) http://www.scotsman.com/news/world/catholic-church-in-la-to-pay-163-325.

Sedge, G. et al. (2012) 'Induced abortion: incident and trends worldwide from 2008 to 1008', *The Lancet* 379: 625–32.

Senlet, P., Cagatay, L. and Matthis, J. (2001) 'Bridging the gap: integrating abortion services with family planning in Turkey', *Int J Family Planning* 27(2) June.

Shadoud, R. (2009) 'The black market of abortion in the Arab World', *Salem News*, 27 March.

Sheridan, M. (2006) 'Forced abortions and genocide in North Korea', *Ontario Consultants on Religious Tolerance*. www.religioustolerance.org/aboforcenk.htm (Accessed 21 February 2013).

Singh, Y. (2004) 'Abortion Nightmare in Nepal', www.news.bbc.co/uk/2/hi/south_asia/397/127.stm (Accessed 16 February 2007).

Singh, S. (2006) 'Hospital admission resulting from unsafe abortion: estimates from 13 developing countries', *The Lancet* 368: 1887–92.

Singson, S. (2008) 'UN World Health Organization circumvents abortion laws in Bangladesh' www.lifenews.com/208/08/21/int-889 (Accessed 30 November 2013).

Sky News (2014) www.news.sky.com/story/1194030. 12 January.

Sokwanele (2012) 'Our ugly secret: abortion in Zimbabwe, illegal but thriving', www-sokwanele.com/node/2374 (Accessed 26 March 2013).

Solo, J. (2008) 'Family planning in Rwanda', *Health International*. www.hindawicom/journals/ijpr/2013/787149 (Accessed 17 April 2013).

Staff reporter (2012) '20,000 women die during abortion each year: report', *New Zimbabwean* 12 April.

Statistics Canada (2007) Induced abortion by area of residence of patients. CANSIM table 106-9013, Catalogue number 822-23-XIE.

Staton, M. (2013) 'Contraceptive methods from the Australian Government', www.ehow.com/list_6852332_cma. (Accessed 29 August 2013).

Steel, C. and Chiarotti, S. (2004) 'With everything exposed: cruelty in post-abortion care in Rosario, Argentina', *Reproductive Health Matters* 12(24): 39–46.

Stone, L. (1977) *The Family, Sex and Marriage in England 1500–1800* London: Weidenfeld and Nicholson.

Storeng, K.T. (2011) *Limited access to post abortion care.* UIO: Institute of Health and Society. www.med.wo.no/.../news2011post-abortion-treatment (Accessed 12 January 2013).

Sung, W.K. (2012) 'Abortion in South Korea:the law and the reality', *Int J Law Policy Family* 3: 278–305.

Takeshita, Y.J., Tan Boon, A. and Arshat, H. (1986) 'Attitudes toward induced abortion', *Malay J of Reproductive Health* (2): 73–90.

Taussig, F.J. (1936) *Abortion – Spontaneous and Induced.* St Louis: C.V. Mosby.

Tavernise, S. (2012) 'Study says meeting contraceptive needs could cut maternal deaths by a third', *New York Times*, 9 July.

Terry, K. (2011) 'Causes and context of sexual abuse of minors by Catholic priests in the US 1950–2010', John Jay College, released 18 May.

Thinh, H.B. (2009) 'Abortion in Vietnam: A Review of Policies and Practices' *Research Centre for Gender, Family, and Environment in Development.* www.arrow.org.my/publications/icpd+is+narrativereport/icpdisvietnam. (Accessed 4 October 2013)

Thompson, D. (2010) 'The Pope and Condoms', *The Daily Telegraph* 23 November, p. 1.

Thwaites, S. (2011) 'Abortion in Malaysia' *Woman's Aid Organization* 13 February. www.wao.org.my/news-details.php?nid=86&ntitle=launch+of+malaysia (Accessed 25 June 2013).

Toussa-Ahossu, A. (1991) 'Contribution a l'etude de la mortalite maternalle dans deux maternities urbaines du Toga'.

Treffers, P.E. (1965*) Abortus en Anticonceptie.* Haarlem: Bohn.

Tremlett, G. (2007) 'Catholic Church fights to keep its grip as Portugal votes on legalizing abortion' *The Guardian* 9 February www.theguardian.cpm/world/2007/feb/09/religion/uk (Accessed 30 September 2013).

Trussell, J. et al. (1980) 'The impact of restricting Medicaid funding for abortion', *Family Planning Perspectives* 12(3): 120–30.

Umutesi, D. (2012) 'Rwanda: Sensitisation on contraceptive use to curb countries high abortion rate' *New Times* (Rwanda's first Daily) www.allafrica.com / stories/201205220068.html (Accessed 3 April 2013).

UNICEF (2006) 'Toward ending female genital mutilation', Press Release, 7 February.

UN Secretariat (2013a) *Abortion Policy: Mali.* New York: UN Population Division.

UN Secretariat (2013b) *Abortion Policy: Somalia.* New York: UN Population Division.

UNFPA (2008) *Egypt: because everyone counts.* New York: UNFPA.

UN (2004) *World Population Monitoring.* New York: UN.

UN (2011) *Madagascar: Tripling Contraceptive Use in Ten Years.* Published in series 'In the News' (internet).

UN (2013) *Abortion in Greece.* www.un.org/esa/population/publications/abortion/ doc/greece.

UN (2014) https://www.un.org/esa/population/publication/abortion/.../Guyana. doc.

UN (2014) www.un.org/esa/population/publications/abortion/doc/chad (Accessed 7 February 2014).

UN (2014) 'Abortion Policy: Tunisia', www.un.org/esa/population/publications/ abortion/doc/tunisia (Accessed 8 February 2014).

Uprety, A. (1998) 'Abortion laws in Nepal', *Body Politic* 8(3).

Usel, R. (2005) 'Young Czechs and the Rhythm Method', Czech Family Planning Association, Prague.

USAID (2012) *The Cost of Family Planning in Kenya.* Published by USAID www. pdf.usaid.gov /pdf.docs/dnadx80 pdf (Accessed 20 March 2013).

Viguerie, R. (1981) *The New Right.* New York: Caroline House.

Vlassoff, M. (2009) *Abortion in Pakistan.* New York: Guttmacher Institute.

Wainer, B. (1972) *Isn't it Nice?* Sydney: Aplan Books.

Walker, A. (2008) 'Saving Nigeria from Risky Abortion', BBC News, April.

Warakamin, S. et al. (2004) 'Induced abortion in Thailand', *Reproductive Health Matters* 12(24): 147–56. (Suppl.).

Warren, M. (2012) 'Argentina's Supreme Court OK's sex slaves', AP, 12 October. www.azcentral.com/strib/world/55072210-68/abortion-court-argentina (Accessed 3 December 2012).

Webb, S. (2000) *Addressing the Problems of Unsafe Abortion.* Watertown, MA: Pathfinder International.

Weinberger, M. (2012) 'Contraceptive use reduces unsafe abortion in Tanzania', www.mariestopes.org/media/nr/2009/10/13/index.html (Accessed 10 March 2013).

Westen, J.H. (2008) 'Guatemala Cardinal on Abortion', 29 August, Life Site News. www.lifesitenews.com/author/jawesten (Accessed 1 November 2012).

White, H. (2011) 'More contraception the solution to Afghan maternal health woes', www.lifesitenews.com/news/.../Afghanistan-maternal-health-needs (Accessed 14 February 2013).

White, H. (2012) 'Uruguayan abortion ban proposal sparks topless protest at cathedral', www.lifesitenews.com/...sparks-topless-feminist-protest-at-cathedral.
Whittaker, A. (2003) *Abortion Law Reform Advocacy in Thailand.* London: Palgrave Macmillan.
WHO (1999) *Abortion in Vietnam.* WHO Geneva.
WHO (2001) Press release, 'Committee on the Elimination of Discrimination against Women'.
WHO (2004) *Unsafe abortion. Global and regional estimates of the incidence of unsafe abortion.* Fourth edition. Geneva.
WHO (2012) World Health Statistics. www.globalhealthfacts.org/data/topic/map.aspx?ind=89 (Accessed 6 July 2013).
WHO (2012a) 'Global and Regional Incidence of Induced Abortion in 2008'.
WHO (2013) Papua New Guinea [Internet].
World Bank (2012) 'World Health Statistics' available at http://www.who.int/gho/publications/world health statistics/2012/ (Accessed 6 June 2013).
World Bank (2012a) 'Contraception in Chad', http://www.tradingeconomics.com/chad/contraception-prevalence-percentage-of-women-aged-15-49
World Bank (2013) 'Unmet need for contraception', http://web.worldbank.org/websight/external/topic/exthethealthunutrition. 25 April.
Women News Network (2011) 16 September, womennewsnetwork.net/2011/09/16/Egypt-abortion-violence.
World Bank (2013) 'Maternal care in Papua New Guinea' (Correspondent S. Mills).
WOW (2011) 'Safe abortion hotline' www.womenonwaves.org/en /pages/3853/dr (Accessed 31 May 2013).
WOW (2012) 'Living in a current where abortion is illegal', Information by email.
WOW (2013) 'Finally men can take the leading role to improve women's health', information direct by email (Accessed 26 September).
Wright, J.W. (2006) *The New York Times Almanac.* Penguin Reference.
Zverina, J. (2005) 'The Czech Republic and Slovakia', *International J of Sexuality.*

Index

Abstinence 129, 192, 195, 198
Albania 6, 20, 22, 23
Afghanistan 2, 6, 53, 54, 58
AIDS (*see* HIV) 8
Albania 6, 20, 22, 23
Algeria 94, 98, 99
Amnesty International 146
Angola 6, 94, 95, 98
Anguilla 142, 143
Antigua 142, 143
Argentina 134–8, 146, 155–68, 199
Armenia 55
Arthur, J. 145
Aspire 164
Australia 5, 6, 169–72, 176
Austria 5, 7, 19, 22, 24–5
Azerbaijan 55

Bahamas 135, 175
Bahrain 55
Banda (bishop)
Bangladesh 53–5, 58, 59
Barbados 131, 135, 138, 141, 144
BPAS 50
Belgium 5, 19, 22, 24, 30, 41, 118, 191
Belarus 19–21
Belize 5, 135
Benin 6, 94
Berer, Marge 15
Bevu, Emily 175
Bhutan 6, 5
Biney 109
Blackburn, Hayley 197
Bolivia 135–6, 138, 139, 168
Bosnia and Herzegovina 19
Bossio, Gara 165
Botha, M.C. 121
Botswana 94, 98
Bourne, Aleck 50, 117, 124, 138, 193
Brandt, W. 28
Brazil 9, 16, 133, 135, 140–2, 168, 199
Brunei 154
Buddhist, Buddhism 14, 15, 70, 73–5, 90
Bulgaria 19, 21, 22
Burkina Faso 6, 94, 99
Bush, George W. 57
Burkina Faso 6, 94, 99
Burundi 6, 94, 95, 101

Cabal Luisa 161
Cameroon 94–5, 101–2
Cambodia 6, 53, 54, 59–60
Canada 5, 177–9, 196
Cape Verde 94
CAWN 152
CEDAW 9, 162
Central African Republic 94–5
Chavez, Hugo 167
Chowdhury Renuka 63
Chad 6, 94, 95, 103
Chile 5, 12, 134–6, 144–6, 168
China 15, 53, 54, 60–3, 75
Choice, Joyce 145
Colombia 6, 16, 133, 135, 147–8, 168, 199
Comoros 94
Conde C.H. 53
Condom(s) 66, 70, 109, 116, 140, 142, 153, 160, 198
Congo 6, 94, 95, 199
Congo DR 103
Costa Rica 135–6, 148, 168
Côte d'Ivoire 94, 104–5
Couriel, A. 166
CRR 162
Croatia 19, 23
Cuba 131, 135, 149, 159, 168
Cyprus 5, 55
Czech Republic 19, 20, 25, 37

Dasgupta, S.M. 61

De Beauvoir, Simone 26
De Marchi, Maria 31–2
Deneuve, Catherine 26
Denmark 5, 19, 20, 52, 170
Dinev, Milka 162
Depo Provera 112
Dominican Republic 133, 135
Dominica 144, 168
Drinan, Robert 9, 200–1

Ecuador 133–5, 154, 196
Egypt 94, 98, 105, 123
Eisenberg 11
El Salvador 3, 135, 136, 146, 149–50, 168
Equatorial Guinea 94
Eritrea 94, 95, 98
Estonia 1, 5, 20, 22
Ethiopia 69, 94–5, 106

Family Planning 2, 6, 24, 35, 66–7, 105, 110, 131, 134, 153, 157, 175
Family Planning Association (FPA) 3, 8, 58–9, 124, 170
Fertility (rates) 8
Foetal abnormality 107–8, 121, 147, 151
FIGO 4
Fiji 5, 26
Finland 5, 19–20, 22, 52
France, French 5, 19, 22, 26–7, 52, 59, 111, 113, 119, 125, 134, 195, 199
Friedman-Rudovsky, J. 139

Gag rule 57
Gallo, L. 166
Gambia 94 97
Genital mutilation 97 120
Georgia 55
Germany 5, 7, 19, 23, 27–8, 41–2, 47, 191 198
Ghana 94, 108
Ghandi, Indira 62
Gomperts Rebecca 37
Greece 5, 7, 19–20, 22, 28–9
Guam 169
Guatemala 5, 131, 135, 152–3
Guinea 6, 95, 109
Guttmacher Institute (GI) 1, 2, 53, 59, 65, 79, 107, 117–18, 121, 133, 141, 148, 158, 182, 184, 186
Guyana 6, 133, 135–6, 144, 153–4, 168

Haiti 133–6, 155–6
Halappanavar Savita 12, 30
Henshaw, S. 20–1, 41, 45, 116–17, 198
Hessini 9, 99, 123
Hindu, Hinduism 10, 14, 49, 58, 129
HIV 35, 62, 75, 85, 102–4, 111, 123, 129, 142, 149, 154, 168, 192, 195, 197, 199
Holland, *see* the Netherlands
Homosexuality 168
Honduras 135, 156–7, 168
Hong Kong 5
Human Rights Watch 103
Hungary 19, 20, 22

Iceland 5, 19, 20, 22
Incest 36, 63, 100, 107–8, 121, 139, 147, 154
In vitro fertilization 4, 36, 38, 148, 201
IPAS 134, 151
IPPF 54–6, 72, 83, 90, 105, 111, 114, 127, 166
Ireland 1, 2, 6, 17, 19–22, 29, 52, 192
India 5, 8, 14–16, 55, 62–4, 82
Indonesia 54, 64–5
Infant mortality rates 20, 99, 136
International Conference on Population and Development (Cairo) (ICPD) 5, 7, 8, 157
Intra Uterine Device (IUD) 2, 4, 24, 60, 66, 70, 87, 89, 115, 187, 193
Iran 9, 55, 65–7
Iraq 55, 67–8
IRIN 93, 110, 116, 174
Israel 5, 17, 53–5, 68–9
Italy 7, 19, 22–3, 42, 44, 134

Jamaica 135, 146, 157–8, 198
Japan 53, 70
Jegasothy, R. 75
Jehu-Appiah, K.S. 109
Jews; Jewish 10, 11, 49, 68–71, 82, 113
Jordan 55

Juarez, F. 158

Kabanda, Iness 130
Kaczynski, J. 36
Kalinde, A. 112
Kane, Gillian 134
Kazakhstan 55, 70, 71
Ketting, Evert 33
Koran, Quran 66
Korea, North 5, 54, 71–2
Korea, South 5, 53, 54, 59, 72–3
Kuwait 5, 54–5, 67, 123

Latvia 19–21
Laos 53–4
Lawson, Agatha 116
Lazaro, F. De S. 140
Lebanon 53, 55
Liberia 6, 94
Libya 94, 103
Lithuania 19–20, 22–3
Luxembourg 5

Mali 6, 113
Malta 191
Malthus (Malthusian) 49
Madagascar 94–5, 111–12
Malaysia 54, 74
Malawi 94, 111–13
Mali 94
Mangom Pastor 113
Manual Vacuum Aspiration (MVA) 9, 14–15, 114, 154, 162
Maputo Treaty (Protocol) 93, 97, 102, 119,
Maternal Mortality 5, 20, 35, 57–8, 60, 77, 89, 98, 106, 120, 124–5, 145, 157
Marx, Karl 49, 60, 149
Mauritania 94
Mauritius 94, 95
Mead, Margaret 175
Mexico; Mexico City 5, 6, 133, 135, 158–9, 168, 191
Mifepristone (RU 486) 15, 171
Millennial Development Goals 8
Misoprostol (Cytotec) 1, 5, 16, 59, 65, 76, 101, 114, 133–4, 140, 148, 151, 157–8, 162
Molina, Ramiro 145
Mongolia 54, 59
Morgentaler, Henry 178
Morocco 5, 94, 113
Mozambique 94–5, 97, 114–15
MSI 51, 58, 75, 78, 83, 91, 109, 111, 125, 171, 173
Muslims; Islam 10, 11, 14, 23, 27, 42, 49, 57, 65–9, 70–1, 73, 99, 101, 103–4, 106, 109, 113, 117, 119, 121, 123, 129, 179
MVA 58–9, 79, 143, 162, 168, 184, 186
Myanmar 54, 56, 75–6

Namibia 94
Nepal 6, 14, 55, 76–8
the Netherlands, Holland 4, 5, 7, 19, 30, 33–4, 41, 143, 161, 191, 195
New Zealand 5, 169, 172–3, 176
Nicaragua 135, 148, 168
Niger 6, 94, 115–16
Nigeria 94, 116
Norway 5–7, 15, 19–20, 22, 35–6
Norwicka, Wanda 38
Nunes, F.E. 154

Offences Against the Person Act 138, 170
Oliver-Miller 173
Oman 54–5
Opinion Polls 137

Pakistan 53–5, 57, 62, 78–9
Panama 135, 160, 168
Papua New Guinea 173–4, 169
Paraguay 135, 168
Paulson, K.D. 13, 14
Peru 5, 16, 113, 134–5, 146, 160–1, 168
Philippines 53–6, 79–81, 199
Pill, the 24–5, 31, 33
PI 109, 161–2, 173
Planned Parenthood 129, 150
Poland 1, 5, 13, 19–20, 23, 36, 47, 191–2,
Pope 10–11, 31, 33, 98, 140, 149, 151, 175, 198–200
Population Action International 7
Portugal, 6, 19, 38–9, 98, 168
Potts, Malcolm 26, 115–16
Prata, G. 98

Pro Life 4, 12, 14, 33, 73, 81, 148, 151, 154
Protestant 23, 27, 29, 103, 144
Puerto Rico 133, 135, 144, 162
Purvis, Dawn 52

Qatar 53–5

Rape 4, 26, 35, 38, 44–5, 50, 58, 63, 74, 84, 99–100, 102–3, 107, 136, 138–9, 141–2, 147–8, 150, 154, 157, 159, 162, 164, 192–3
Rhythm method 25, 74
Roa Monica 147
Romania 4, 19–20, 22, 39–40
Rossier, C. 100
Roth, Kenneth 159
Russian Federation 5, 19–23, 40–3, 47, 57, 49
Rwanda 94–5, 118–19, 124

St Lucia 6, 135, 144
Safe period 25
Sanger, Margaret 163
Samoa 169, 175–6
Saudi Arabia 55, 81
Schuster, S. 102
Scotland 15
Senegal 94, 119–20
Serbia 19–20, 22
Seychelles 5, 94
Sharif, S. 110
Shaw, Dorothy 1, 4
Shintoism 15, 70
Sierra Leone 94, 97
Sikh 10, 15, 49
Singapore 5, 53, 170
Sai, Frederick 131
Schneider, Romy 28
Slovakia 19, 20, 25
Somalia 94–5, 120
South Africa 5–6, 9, 120–2, 131
South Sudan 122–3
Soviet Union, *see* Russia
Spain, Spanish 5, 7, 19, 39, 44–6, 149, 161, 168, 195, 199
Sri Lanka 55, 83–4
Sterilization 24, 62
Sudan 94, 123
Swaziland 6, 94
Sweden 5, 7, 19, 20, 22, 46–7, 52, 170
Switzerland 4, 6, 19, 191
Syria 55, 84–5

Tajikistan 55
Tanzania 94–5, 124–5
Thailand 54, 85–6
Timor Leste 6, 169, 174
Togo 6, 94, 125
Trinidad and Tobago 135, 144, 163
Trudeau, Pierre 177
Tunisia 5, 94, 97–9, 126–7
Turkey 53, 86–7
Turkmenistan 53, 55

Uganda 6, 94–5, 127–8, 199
UNICEF 136
Ukraine 19–20, 23, 47
United Arab Emirates 5, 55
United Nations 9, 17, 63, 58, 64, 69, 93, 154–5, 161–2, 174
United Nations Population Fund (UNFPA) 59
Uruguay 6, 133, 135–6, 164–5, 168
Uzbekistan 55, 83
Uzel Radim 19

Vanuatu 169, 175
Vasectomy 62, 66
Vatican 24, 136, 191
Venezuela 134–5, 146, 164, 166, 168
Verna, St Rose Greaves 164
Veil, Simone 26
Vietnam 53–4, 89–90
Virgin Islands 135–6

White, S. 112
Withdrawal 25
World Bank 175
World Health Organization 1
WOW 16, 37, 109, 134, 150

Yemen 55, 90

Zambia 94–5, 129
Zimbabwe 5, 16, 94–5, 131

For Product Safety Concerns and Information please contact our EU representative GPSR@taylorandfrancis.com Taylor & Francis Verlag GmbH, Kaufingerstraße 24, 80331 München, Germany

Batch number: 10725973

Printed by Printforce, the Netherlands